# ROOTS OF CHINESE CULTURE AND MEDICINE

Wei Tsuei

ACCHS Series: No. 1

Chinese Culture Books Co.
Oakland, California, U.S.A.

Library of Congress catalog card number: 89-51907

ISBN: 0-9625156-0-4

Printed in the United States of America.

10 9 8 7 6 5 4 3 2 1

中國文化

醫藥之根

肖巍

自署

# Preface

As a master of traditional Chinese martial arts, medicine, philosophy and culture, I am trying to create a new synthesis of East and West. This book introduces the Western reader to the essential aspects of Chinese culture and philosophy and presents my ideas about the Taichi philosophy.

Emphasizing that Chinese philosophy and culture are the roots of traditional Chinese medicine, the book begins with a discussion of culture in general and Chinese culture in particular. Along with this comes a brief explanation of the *I Ching (The Book of Change)*. Next, the book provides an introduction to the two greatest Chinese philosophers, Confucius and Lao-tzu, and then turns to a discussion of Buddhism and Christianity, the major religions brought into China from other cultures. Following this, an examination of Zen focuses on the ways it blends Indian Buddhism with Chinese Confucianism and Taoism. Then follows an overview of Western medicine and a broad outline of traditional Chinese medicine. The last chapter synthesizes the general Taichi philosophy and points out just a few of its many applications.

This book is based on my doctoral dissertation at the San Francisco College of Acupuncture in 1984, and my classroom lectures to students of Chinese medicine at The Academy of Chinese Culture and Health Sciences from 1984 to 1989. In the classroom, my aim is to teach students to understand the theory and practice of traditional Chinese medicine from its roots in culture and philosophy, with Yin Yang theory at its core. However, this book is not only intended for students in a traditional Chinese medical college, but for anyone with an interest in the subjects of Chinese culture, philosophy and healing arts. Medicine is an aspect of culture; indeed, it is an aspect of vital importance and broad interest to all. A person whose interests lie in the field of medicine can benefit from the culturally enhanced view of Chinese traditional medicine presented here, while one more interested in human culture can view a cross-section of Chinese culture through these materials. Thus, I hope this book will reach a more general audience.

It is my belief that the contemporary practitioner of Chinese medicine can best meet the physical, mental and spiritual needs of his or her patients by integrating Chinese medicine with Taichi Chuan, Chi Kung and meditation. This must be achieved in the context of traditional Chinese culture and philosophy. Indeed, all humanity can benefit from the integration of culture, philosophy and medicine, and it is my hope that this integration will reach the widest possible range of people. The Taichi circle, embracing both Yin and Yang, is the major topic of this book and may serve as a comprehensive model for medicine, philosophy, and culture.

Students of Chinese culture always come back to a subject discussed in China for over 5,000 years: Yin and Yang. Just as our shadow never leaves us, our spiritual lives can never be separated from our material pursuits and interpersonal relationships. I therefore advise my students, as well as the readers of this book, to devote themselves to a deep study of the Yin Yang balance and the Taichi circle, the relative and the absolute, the whole rather than merely the parts.

I would like to acknowledge my gratitude to those staff members and students of the Taoist Center and the Academy of Chinese Culture and Health Sciences who gave their invaluable assistance in the research, editing, and production of this book.

# About the Author

Born in Wuxing County, Zhejiang Province, China, into a family that had practiced traditional Chinese medicine for several generations, Wei Tsuei learned traditional Chinese medicine and martial arts from boyhood, in the Chinese way. He then studied Chinese philosophy and meditation, Taichi Chuan (Yang Family Style, 127 movements) and Xiu Shen (the Tao of self-cultivation). The sixth-generation successor of traditional Chinese Xiu Shen Tao and Chi Kung from the school of Golden Elixir, he completed these studies in his middle years and started giving instruction at that time.

For the past thirty years, Shifu (the respectful form of address for a teaching master) has taught meditation as well as Taichi Chuan and other martial arts in both Taiwan and the United States. In Taiwan, he served as instructor and director at the Chinese Academy of Taichi Chuan, consultant for the Taipei Association for the Chinese Martial Arts and the Municipal Government of Taipei and instructor at the Chinese Martial Arts Society at the University of Taiwan.

In the sixties, Shifu (or Sifu) completed his formal training in acupuncture, established his own medical practice and also taught Chinese medicine at Tai Tung Clinic of Chinese Medicine and the Quang Wah Acupuncture Clinic in Taipei. He acted as consultant at the Taipei Academy of Acupuncture before coming to the United States in 1972. Consistent with his professional commitment to continue studying throughout his career, Shifu earned one of the first American doctorates in Oriental Medicine.

Believing that the traditional Chinese doctor ministers not only to individuals but to society as well, Shifu founded the Taoist Center in Oakland, California in 1973. Combining the best of China's ancient culture with American science and technology,

Taoist Center students learn traditional Chinese methods of developing good health and character. The Center includes an acupuncture clinic and has offered classes in Taichi Chuan, Chi Kung, Push Hands, Taichi Sword, Taichi meditation and cooking with herbs to over 3,000 pupils.

Building on the Taoist Center, Shifu established the Academy of Chinese Culture and Health Sciences (ACCHS) in 1984. Approved in 1985 by the California Acupuncture Examining Committee, this college educates students in all cultural aspects of Chinese medicine, preparing graduates to become licensed as acupuncturists and practitioners of traditional Chinese medicine.

Various articles have introduced the Taoist Center, ACCHS and Shifu to American society:

Lonnie Isabel, "Eastbay Gets Its First Acupuncture College," *The Tribune* (Oakland, CA), August 12, 1984; Christine Keyser, "Acupuncturist Keeps His Patients on Pins and Needles," *San Francisco Examiner*, February 27, 1985; Roberta Alexander, "Learning Where to Put Those Needles: East Meets West at Acupuncture Academy Where Disciplines Are Mixed," *San Francisco Examiner*, December 4, 1985; Marsha Newman, "Vignette of a Taichi Master," *New Realities*, January/February, 1985: p. 5; William Rodarmor, "Master of Meridians: Martial Artist, Teacher, and Healer, Sifu Tsuei Wei Is Living Testimony to 5,000 years of Chinese Culture," *Yoga Journal*, March/April, 1986: pp. 30–32; Sarah Vitale, Ed., "Tsuei, Wei," *Who's Who in California*, 19th ed., The Who's Who Historical Society, 1990, p. 563.

What Shifu Tsuei has to say in this book is deceptively simple. Its value can best be appreciated when one realizes that application of his philosophy can unify into one whole the physical, mental and spiritual levels of an individual's life or of a culture's life.

> Editorial Group,
> Taoist Center and
> ACCHS

# Contents

# List of Illustrations

# Notes on Romanization of Chinese Characters

The pinyin style of romanization is used in this book except for terms and names that are well known in other spellings. The following list shows some of these familiar words as they are used in this book and their pinyin romanization. The first time each term appears in the book, it is given in both styles. Romanization in direct quotations and references from other publications vary, and may use either pinyin, Wade-Giles or other systems of romanization.

| Wade-Giles or other system | Pinyin style |
|---|---|
| Zen | Chan |
| Tao, Taoism, Taoist | Dao, Daoism, Daoist |
| Tao Te Ching | Dao De Jing |
| Confucius | Kongzi |
| Lao-tzu | Laozi |
| Taichi | Taiji |
| Taichi Chuan | Taiji Quan |
| Chi | Qi |
| Chi Kung | Qi Gong |
| I Ching | Yi Jing |

# CHAPTER 1
# Culture and Taichi Philosophy

## The Concepts of Taichi Philosophy and Culture

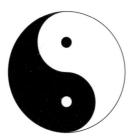

Even in the Western world many people are familiar with the diagram above: the Taichi symbol. On the surface, it looks very simple: a Yin, a Yang, and a circle. Yet, this symbol represents a deep and universal theory: Yin, Yang, and Taichi circle (or 1, 2, and 3—Three into One). It is the core of the Taichi philosophy. $E = mc^2$. What could be simpler than an equation with only three terms? Without knowing the problems and obstacles faced by thousands of scientific minds before him and with little or no knowledge of the intricate relationship between energy and matter symbolized by the formulation, anyone looking at Einstein's three terms may ask such a question. Similarly, Americans unfamiliar with the long and venerable philosophical tradition from which the Taichi symbol has been borrowed, when asked what

1

it means, would probably say the circle symbolizes the result aimed at in the practice of **Taichi Chuan** (Taiji Quan), a form of disciplined exercise leading to a balanced relationship between mind and body.

The art of Taichi Chuan, however, is but one practical application of a philosophical tradition which, for thousands of years, has studied and examined our world's myriad manifestations of the relationship between permanence and change. Just as Einstein's expression finally distills a universal principle with which generations of scientific genius have grappled, the Taichi symbol elegantly encapsulates all that we can and cannot know about ourselves and our universe.

Simply stated, the One—the Taichi circle—encircles the Two: the black Yin and the white Yang, always becoming each other, always beginning each other, each always containing a bit of the other, always moving towards the balanced circle. It is simple to say, less simple to practice, and even less simple to attain in a short time.

Slowly and gently, then, this book attempts to unfold Taichi philosophy to the reader as the reader unfolds to Taichi. [In this book Taichi is not the abbreviated form of Taichi Chuan, or other Taichi exercises. It stands for the Taichi philosophy, Taichi theory, or Taichi model, all of which can be used interchangeably.] As the book and reader unfold the essence of each other, become each other, begin each other, both will move simultaneously toward and within the balance of Taichi. For only in the movement comes its understanding.

In Chinese, **Taichi** (Taiji) means "supreme ultimate." It consists of two Chinese characters "Tai" and "Chi." The word **Tai** means highest or greatest; **Chi** can also mean high, supreme, or the utmost pole or extreme. The Taichi symbol, or Tachi model, represents two relative factors, **Yin** and **Yang**, and their relation to the original One, the absolute whole, the Taichi circle.

The earliest existing source in which Yin and Yang were described is the *I Ching* (*Yi Jing*, *The Book of Change*, see detailed in Chapter 3): "A Yin and a Yang are called **Tao** (Dao)," and "The Tao that set up heaven and earth is called Yin Yang." The

Taichi philosophy, which emerged from the earliest roots of Chinese culture, is present in the ancient philosophical and medical texts, as well as in the Taoist and Confucian classics. This theory has colored all of Chinese thinking and can be used as a tool to understand aspects of the world and ourselves on any level. It is the major topic of this book.

## Culture and Life

Culture is a very broad subject, and the word culture has had and retains a number of meanings. Generally speaking, all activities not resulting solely from animal instinct, all activities belonging specifically to people, are a part of culture. Thus, human beings are animals with culture.

Culture is deeply intertwined with individual human lives, in that these individual lives make up the whole which is culture. If culture is a circle, the life of an individual is one of the points on its circumference. Without each point there would be no circle, and without the circle no individual points. Thus, culture and the individual life cannot be ranked one above the other, for they are two aspects of the same thing. With regard to culture and life, it makes no sense to ask "which came first, the chicken or the egg."

Culture is the total way of life of the human being. Culture, therefore, varies with every group or society, depending on what its historical experience has been; it represents the distinctive way of life of a group of people, their complete design for living. A particular culture—one developed by a particular society—would consist of the patterns of learned behavior shared by the members of that society. This would include attitudes, ideas, values, knowledge, skills, and material objects. We can identify as many cultures as there are societies.[1]

Culture exists through constant development or change rather than mere preservation of tradition. In Chinese, the two characters making up the word for culture are **Wen** and **Hua**. Wen means civilization, and Hua means change or transformation.[2]

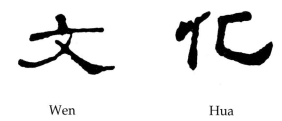

Wen                    Hua

There is an ancient Chinese saying which states: "Immortality governs change." Change is the only constant. The transformations of culture may involve barely noticeable departures or revolutionary changes. Culture can be divided into three broad categories, or three levels.

1. The first level of culture: the aspect pertaining to material goods, or people in relation to things.
2. The second level of culture: the aspect pertaining to society, or people in relation to people.
3. The third level of culture: the aspect pertaining to spirit, or people's hearts in relation to people's hearts.[3]

The first level deals with the basic necessities of survival such as food, clothing and shelter. The second level of culture deals with the dynamics of social interaction. The third level of culture deals with the human heart. A Chinese proverb states "People's hearts are different, just as no two faces are alike," yet individual hearts and minds do have something in common. The sole desire of the heart is to expand: we have a natural desire to express our thoughts and feelings to others. A shared thought or a feeling becomes a heart-to-heart link, a gift to others. This giving from the heart strengthens the thought and deepens the feeling. Only through heart-to-heart sharing can we eventually unify the body of mankind. The heart is the strongest element in human culture. It is the heart which inspires, reaches out, accumulates, changes, enjoys. On this level, we understand that joy, anger, grief and pleasure are feelings all people share. To overindulge in the material level spoils the appetite; on the political level, power corrupts. By providing sufficient material goods and developing political stability, we can inspire the exchange of thoughts and feelings between hearts and minds. This will give new hope to mankind. Keep in mind that the three aspects are not linear; cultures include all three levels simultaneously. In terms of the Taichi philosophy, we could call the first and second levels of culture Yin and Yang, and the third level the Taichi circle. The third level, like the circumference of the circle, combines and transcends the relative factors, Yin and Yang, or the lower levels of culture.

Yin and Yang are relative concepts; that is to say, they reveal themselves through contrast. Considering problems from the point of view of Yin and Yang allows one to keep greater balance, while a culture lacking the perspective of Yin and Yang will fall into one-sidedness and arrogance. Yin and Yang are the vital core of China's culture. Still, the Chinese also bear in mind that it is not good to play too many games with Yin and Yang. For example, Chinese has the sayings "Yin yi tou, Yang yi tou" (one face in Yin, one face in Yang—hiding one's true intentions), and "Yin Yang guai qi" (strange Yin Yang airs, acting weird).

Taichi philosophy emphasizes Yin and Yang balanced within the Taichi circle. People who are conscious of this level of Yin Yang balance can better align their individual hearts and actions to form a harmonious whole, like the Taichi symbol.

## Culture and Healing

Culture itself has life. By saying this, we mean that culture can be viewed as a growing, changing, learning and interacting organism. A culture, too, can be healthy or afflicted with disease; a culture, too, can be born, grow old and die out; a culture, too, can have a relationship with other cultures.

Both cultures and individual lives can get sick and require healing. Internally healthy people and cultures are less susceptible to disease. For a person or a culture to be healthy, the development of material, interpersonal and spiritual levels should be parallel and balanced. Individuals, societies, or countries lacking in sound spirit will be plagued by illness. Addictions to money, power, drugs, or excessive sex can result in culturally-based diseases.

The medical arts of China are valuable because they developed within a culture that spans more than 5,000 years of written history, covers a vast geographical area, and contains the world's largest population. Instead of experimenting on laboratory animals, Chinese doctors have tested their hypotheses by observing living human beings. Over centuries of empirical study and research, they have continued to keep what is good and useful and to discard what is not valid. Chinese medicine comes from the same intangible energy as its culture, which has kept China alive through geographic and political change. It is the continuous growth of the culture that has allowed the medical arts to mature.

Ultimately, no matter what culture we speak of, Eastern or Western, those who are able to cure illness and heal people are good doctors. Major cultural transformation is now within reach for Americans. The blooming of many different coexisting cultures will be beneficial to all. Composed of people from a diversity of backgrounds, the United States of America is a country with an excellent opportunity to integrate different cultures, to one day became the "United States of Cultures." It will be a very long and difficult process. When discussing world problems, it is important to start from a cultural perspective and to look at the long term patterns and effects. We need to face the deep questions of our lives to develop a healthy world culture, a new and ideal united culture inherited from the past and working for the future.

# CHAPTER 2
# Chinese Nationality, History, and Culture

This chapter is a very brief summary which cannot give more than a basic background and a general understanding of China's five-thousand-year-old culture. Understanding the essence of Chinese history is important in understanding the Taichi philosophy, since they originated and grew out of the same sources. The table on the following page briefly outlines the dynasties and key events.[4]

The cultural prehistory of China is of unknown antiquity. In 1927, geologists of the Academia Sinica discovered human head bones at Choukkoudian (Zhoukoudian). After examination by anthropologists of various countries, the bones were identified as human remains dating back 578,000 years.[5] Choukkoudian is situated at the lower reaches of the Yellow River (Huang Ho, or Huanghe) Valley about a hundred miles southwest of Beijing (Peking), so the earliest Chinese people found there were named Peking Man (Sinanthropus Pekinensis). They were the remote ancestors of the Chinese.

The present Chinese culture is a continuation of a major stream in the gradual evolution of mankind. The ancestors of the Chinese people have been in written historical evidence in Asia for thousands of years, while most other civilizations that old have disintegrated, leaving only relics. The time from the chaos at the beginning of the world to the time of Huang Di was the period

7

| Dynasties Approx. Dates | People and Events |
|---|---|
| **Legendary Period** (2852–2197 B.C.) | |
| | Fu Xi—Yin Yang |
| | Shen Nong  *Herbalist* |
| | Huang Di  *Yellow Emperor* |
| | *Nei Jing* |
| **Primitive Dynasties** (2197–221 B.C.) | |
| Xia [Hsia] (1994–1523 B.C.) | "Great Flood" brought under control |
| Shang [Yin] (1523–1027 B.C.) | Casting of Bronze. |
| | Oracle Bones of Yin. |
| Zhou [Chou] (1027–221 B.C.) | Lao-tzu, Confucius, Mencius. |
| **Ancient Dynasties** (221 B.C.-618 A.D.) | |
| Qin [Ch'in] (221–207 B.C.) | Great Wall built, languages standardized. |
| Han (207 B.C.-220 A.D.) | Confucianism established. |
| | Buddhism introduced (64 A.D.). |
| Three Kingdom (220–265) | |
| Jin [Chin] (265–420) | |
| North & South (420–589) | Buddhism well developed. |
| Sui (589–618) | |
| **Medieval Dynasties** (618–1368 A.D.) | |
| Tang [T'ang] (618–905) | Arts & literature develop, |
| | printing invented. |
| Five Dynasties (905–960) | |
| Song [Sung] (960–1279) | Neo-Confucian philosophy. |
| Yuan [Mongol] (1280–1368) | Marco Polo to China. |
| **Modern Dynasties** (1368–1911 A.D.) | |
| Ming (1368–1644) | Painting, industry, all arts flourish. |
| Qing [Ch'ing, Manchu] (1644–1911) | Opium War. T'aiping Rebellion. |

in Chinese history known as the legendary.[6] There is no reliable recorded history of this period, but descriptions may be found in ancient books.

In Chinese mythology, the world began with Pan Ku (Pan Gu), the creator, who was followed by the divine and semidivine beings. The divine beings were the "San Huang" (Three Emperors): Tian Huang (Emperor of Heaven), Di Huang (Emperor of Earth), and Ren Huang (Emperor of Man). The semi-divine beings were four cultural heroes who are credited with having first taught the Chinese people the various arts of civilization. It is said that You Cao (Shi, meaning Master, or Mister) taught people to build dwellings of wood; Sui Ren (Shi) to make fire by boring wood; Fu Xi (Shi) to fish and hunt with nets and to raise cattle; and Shen Nong (Shi) to cultivate grain with hoes and to cure sickness with herbs.

Fu Xi and Shen Nong are very important. Fu Xi is credited with the invention of Yin Yang and their symbols.

Yin                              Yang

Fu Xi realized that everything is constantly changing, and created the symbols ▬▬ and ▬ ▬ to represent change. These ideas developed into the classic *I Ching* (*Yi Jing, The Book of Change*, see Chapter 3). Shen Nong is said to have invented the wooden plow and methods of farming, which moved the population away from a nomadic lifestyle. This had great impact on the culture. He is also credited with having been the first to personally taste and use Chinese herbs. The earlist extant Chinese pharmacology book, dating from the 1st and 2nd centuries A.D., *Shen Nong's Canon of Herbs*, is attributed to his great name.

The legendary figures were followed by the era of the "Wu Di" (Five Emperors)—the Yellow Emperor (Huang Di), Emperor Chuan Hsu (Zhuan Xu), Emperor Ku, Emperor Yao, and Emperor

Shun. Huang Di (2698–2589 B.C.) is best known to students of Chinese medicine in association with the *Huangdi Nei Jing* (*The Yellow Emperor's Canon of Internal Medicine*).

The ancestors of the Chinese people lived along the Yellow River, and like all nations, their lives were formed around the natural forces and features of their environment. By using local vegetation and developing methods of production, they met their needs for survival. In time, their habits evolved into distinctive traditions. In the early stage of development, people lived in migratory tribes. One of these tribes has come to be known as the Xia Zu, meaning the Xia race, also called the Hua Zu. The name became Hua Xia Min Zu, or the Chinese nation. The legendary leader of this group was Huang Di, who defeated Chih Yu (Chi You), chieftain of another tribe, in a battle around 2670 B.C. The battle was decisive, and ever since then the Hua Zu people have been living in China. Thus, Chinese like to refer to themselves as descendants of Huang Di.

During the era of Huang Di, there was progress in the methods of accumulation and distribution of surplus goods. The most important culture of this period is known as the Yangshao Culture. Another Huang Di Neolithic culture, called Long Shan, followed the Yangshao Period. This culture was more advanced than that of the Yangshao Period and probably knew the use of the wheel in transportation. According to the *I Ching* and *Shi Ji* (*Historical Annals*), people in the Long Shan Period knew how to carve a canoe from a log and to split a board into an oar. The Huang Di era yielded many innovations which had far-reaching influence on later generations, such as the study of astronomy, a progressive farming system called "Jingtian," the invention of pictographs by Cang Jie, and the invention of the compass, called the "south-pointing carriage."

Yao, Shun, and Shun's successor Yu were considered model emperors with exceptional wisdom and virtue. During Yao's time, there were the establishment of government positions and rites, cultural emphasis on the importance of people rather than deities, further development of agriculture, and an orderly transfer of power through the appointment of a successor to the throne. During the Yu Period, the so-called "great flood" was brought under control. Establishing the Xia Dynasty, Yu left his throne to his son, thus originating the system of hereditary succession to the position of emperor, usually by the emperor's son.

In important excavations between 1979 and 1986 in the west of Liaoning province, Chinese archaeologists discovered a great deal of reliable evidence of the early "Hongshan (Red Mountain) Civilization." The discoveries included a Goddess temple and sacrificial altar which were built over 5,000 years ago. This was the first archaeological evidence of Chinese culture before the Xia Dynasty (the first known Chinese dynasty).

Shang, or Yin, was the second dynasty, lasting from the 16th century B.C. to the 11th century B.C. During the Shang Dynasty, a bronze culture evolved. The discovery of thousands of inscribed bones and tortoise shells in An-yang, Honan (Henan) province, between 1928 and 1937, has given historians firm evidence regarding the Shang Dynasty.

Zhou (Chou) was the third dynasty. With this dynasty, China entered a feudal system of government. Most Chinese laws, political institutions, art, and literature can be traced back to roots in the Zhou Dynasty, during which time the population greatly increased. The Zhou Dynasty can be divided into Western Zhou (1111 B.C.–771 B.C.) and Eastern Zhou (770 B.C.–221 B.C.). Eastern Zhou can be further divided into the Spring-and-Autumn Period (770 B.C.–476 B.C.) and the Warring States Period (475 B.C.–221 B.C.). During these eras, culture flourished as a response to the demands of the times. Beginning in the Zhou Dynasty, China had written historical records and books. It was a very rich and important age in Chinese history; this era saw the beginnings of philosophical schools (Confucianism, Taoism, Mohism, Legalism, etc., called "zhuzi baijia," literally "one hundred various schools"), and medicine.

After the Zhou Dynasty, in the Qin (255 to 206 B.C.) and Han (206 B.C. to 220 A.D.) Dynasties, the boundaries of the Chinese nation extended to the south to cover such present provinces as Fujian, Guangdung, Yunnan, and the present nation of Vietnam. To the east was the China Sea, to the north the desert of Mongolia, and to the west the Pamir Plateau. The Han people had a predominant impact on culture, having in common the same "blood" or genetics, language, writing, customs and habits. When foreign tribes invaded (the Mongols ruled from 1280 to 1368 A.D. and the Manchus from 1644 to 1912), the conquerors could not dominate the Han and were eventually assimilated by them.

Qin Shihuang (the First Emperor of Qin) standardized the written Chinese language—the Chinese characters. This has been a very important factor in the extraordinarily long survival of Chinese culture. The thousands of written characters or ideograms that Chinese use singly or in pairs to represent words have changed little over the last 2,000 years, and this written language has been a great unifying force in Chinese history and culture. Although local languages and dialects hinder spoken contacts between people from different regions, written characters are uniform throughout China. Japan and Korea have also used Chinese characters in their written languages for many centuries.

The third level of culture in China, as well as the art of traditional Chinese medicine, was well developed by the end of the Han Dynasty. Confucianism had entered the mainstream of Chinese culture, Taoism as both philosophy and religion had been established, and Buddhism had been introduced into China. The Han Dynasty was one of the peaks in the cycle of Chinese culture.

An excavation in 1972 outside the city of Changsha, in Hunan Province, revealed much information about Han Dynasty culture. The site, identified as being 2,100 years old, contained a tomb consisting of six layers of coffins placed one within another, tightly packed in charcoal sealed with clay. The innermost coffin contained the well-preserved embalmed body of a fifty-year-old woman. The clay seals and inscriptions in ink on the burial accessories were those of the Marquis of Ta, a hereditary title

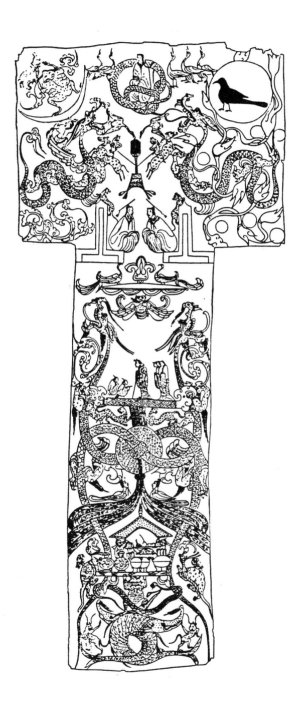

conferred by the Emperor Hui in 193 B.C. and withdrawn in the fourth generation. The body is surmised to be that of the wife of the first Marquis of Ta, a petty noble with a fief containing about 700 households. More than one thousand burial accessories were found, including lacquerware, wooden figurines, bamboo and wooden utensils, pottery, grain, foodstuffs, specially made funerary objects, and many exquisitely woven silk fabrics. The most valuable of these is a painted silk shroud that draped the innermost coffin.[7]

The painting is divided into three parts: the upper portion represents the realm of god or heaven, the middle depicts the human realm, the lower part shows the realm of hell. This ancient concept of Heaven, Earth and Man relates to the three levels of culture. The top images symbolize Yin and Yang with paintings of the sun holding a crow, and the moon holding a toad and a rabbit. The Five Elements are depicted as five birds, corresponding with a legend that the earliest form of acupuncture was a pecking bird. The middle part of the shroud shows what is probably a scene from the daily life of the wife of the Marquis. The bottom part of the shroud shows scenes of sea and land, demons and a dragon. This shroud comes from a time when Yin and Yang were known, but before the idea of the Taichi circle, which came 1,000 years later.

# CHAPTER 3
# I Ching
# (The Book of Change)
# and Its Impact

What does the word **Ching** (Jing) mean? The sages and people of virtue in ancient China recorded their valuable scholarship and thoughts on the principles of living in classical writings. Jing means a classic, a most eminent book that can help people to open their minds. Examples of classics include the Fo Jing (the Buddhist Sutra) and the Sheng Jing (the Bible). The noted ancient Chinese classics known as the Wu Jing (Five Classics) include five books (see Chapter 4), of which the *I Ching* has the prime place. In China, where knowledge and learning are concerned, one cannot do without a discussion of the *I Ching*.

What, then, is **I** (Yi)? In the character Yi we can see abstract pictorial representations of the sun and moon. In their constant movement, the sun and moon come close to signifying the idea of eternity, as in the expression "change is the only constant."

| Sun | Moon | Sun & Moon | Yi | Yin/Yang |
|------|------|------------|-----|----------|
| (Yang) | (Yin) | (Yin and Yang) | | |

15

The word for sun, "Ri," also means male (Yang), and the word for moon, "Yue," means female (Yin). Put together, they become the word Yi, which includes the characteristics of Yin and Yang. Combined with other characters, Yi creates expanded meanings of the concept of change. For example, "Jian Yi" means simple or easy, "Bian Yi" means changing, and "Bu Yi" means complex. All these are characteristics of change.

Yi means:

| | | |
|---|---|---|
| simple | (Jian Yi) | Taiji |
| changeable | (Bian Yi) | absolute |
| complex | (Bu Yi) | relative |

We can relate Jian Yi to Taichi in that both basic principles are profoundly simple, Bian Yi to the absolute in being constantly changing, Bu Yi to the relative, very complicated. As in the Taichi diagram, Yin and Yang are dynamic, balance creates ease, and the circle is absolute.

The *I Ching* is a book about the change and permanence of the universe. The universe is in movement or transformation at every moment. Life itself is a process of never-ending change from birth to death. All creatures have life. The beginnings of a life are given by the mother and father. Growth depends on the assistance of heaven and earth, the spiritual and physical. *I Ching* is an attempt to find reliable rules for nature, and for human life in relation to changes in the universe, so that people might live better.

The *I Ching* grew out of the ancient practice of divination.[8] As a text, it is valued by the Confucians and Taoists alike. It is divided into the texts and commentaries. The texts consist of discussions of sixty-four hexagrams. These hexagrams are based on the Eight Trigrams. Each of the Trigrams consists of three lines: divided ▬ ▬ and undivided ▬▬▬ , the divided representing Yin and the undivided representing Yang. Each of these eight corresponds to a direction, a natural element, a moral quality, etc.

Each of the Eight Trigrams is combined with another, one above the other, thus making sixty-four hexagrams. The following illus-

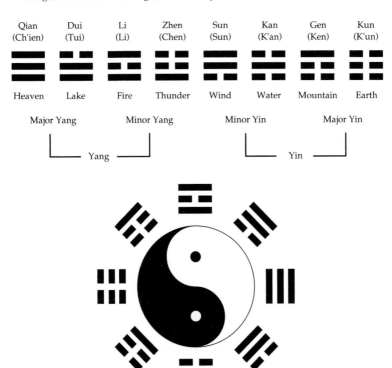

| Qian (Ch'ien) | Dui (Tui) | Li (Li) | Zhen (Chen) | Sun (Sun) | Kan (K'an) | Gen (Ken) | Kun (K'un) |
|---|---|---|---|---|---|---|---|
| Heaven | Lake | Fire | Thunder | Wind | Water | Mountain | Earth |

Major Yang   Minor Yang   Minor Yin   Major Yin

Yang   Yin

tration shows how the sixty-four hexagrams are generated line-by-line, from Yin and Yang alternating one by one, two by two, four by four, and so on.

These hexagrams symbolize all possible situations. For example, as discussed in Chapter 10, the 64th hexagram "Wei Ji" (Before Completion), with the fire trigram over the water trigram, symbolizes what is not yet completed.[9] (See the illustration on the following page.)

The *I Ching* is a very complicated book. It consists of the following parts:

The Text

Section I      Hexagrams Nos. 1–30
Section II     Hexagrams Nos. 31–64

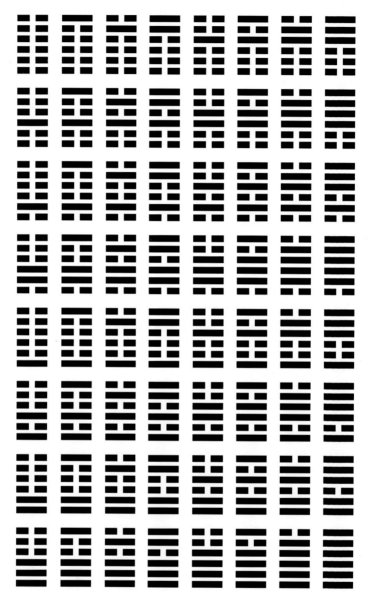

line 1: 1 Yin, 1 Yang　　　line 4:　8 Yin,　8 Yang
line 2: 2 Yin, 2 Yang　　　line 5: 16 Yin, 16 Yang
line 3: 4 Yin, 4 Yang　　　line 6: 32 Yin, 32 Yang

The following explanations come after each hexagram:
(1) the "kua-tz'u," the explanation of the text of the whole hexagram
(2) the "yao-tz'u," the explanation of the component lines (Each hexagram has 6 lines.)
(3) the "chuan," the commentary on "kua-tz'u"
(4) the "hsiang," the abstract meaning of "kua-tz'u" and "yao-tz'u"
(5) the "wen-yen" or commentary on the first two hexagrams (ch'ien and k'un) to stress their philosophical and ethical meaning

The Appendixes
(6) the great appendix ("hsi-tz'u")
Section I    Chapters 1–12
Section II   Chapters 1–12
(7) the remarks on certain trigrams Chapters 1–10
(8) the remarks on the order of the hexagrams
(9) the miscellaneous remarks on the hexagrams

Numbers (3), (4), (5), (6), (7), (8), and (9), with their sections, form the "Shiyi" ("Ten Wings") of the book. The most important parts are the texts, (1) and (2), the commentary (5), the great appendix (6), and the remarks (7).

Tradition has ascribed the Eight Trigrams to the legendary ruler Fu Xi , the sixty-four hexagrams to King Wen (1171–1122 B.C.), and the two texts to King Wen or to Duke Zhou (d. 1094 B.C.). The "Ten Wings" are traditionally ascribed to Confucius (Kongzi). Most scholars have rejected this attribution, but they are not in agreement about when and by whom the book was produced. Most probably it is a product of many minds over a long period of time, from the fifth or sixth century B.C. to the third or fourth century B.C.[10]

The Ten Wings consist of commentaries on the hexagrams as a whole (kua-tz'u), explanations of the six component lines (yao-tz'u), abstract meanings given to the hexagrams and lines (hsiang), commentaries on the first two hexagrams stressing their philosophical and ethical meaning (wen-yen), the Great Appendix (hsi-ts'u), and remarks on certain of the trigrams, remarks on the order of the hexagrams, and further miscellaneous remarks. The most important parts are the texts explaining the hexagrams and their component lines, the discussions on ch'ien and k'un, the great appendix and the remarks on certain trigrams. These sections have been the basis of much philosophical speculation.

The following are some frequently cited passages from the *I Ching* which relate to Yin and Yang, Three into One and Taichi:

> Therefore in the system of Yi (Change) there is the "Tai Ji" (Great Ultimate). It generates the "Liang Yi" (Two Modes, i.e. Yin and Yang). The Two Modes generate the "Si Xiang" (Four Forms, i.e. major and minor Yin and Yang). The Four Forms generate the "Ba Gua" (Eight Trigrams). The Eight Trigrams determine good and evil fortunes. And good and evil fortunes produce the great business [of life].[11]

From the One, two and then many are generated. Life is a process of interplay among the infinite and constantly changing manifestations of Yin and Yang. This concept is essential to Taoist philosophy, and is beautifully expressed in Lao-tzu's *Tao Te Ching* (Laozi's *Dao De Jing*), discussed in Chapter 5.

> The successive movement of Yin and Yang constitutes the Tao (Way). What issues from the Tao is good, and that which realizes it is the individual nature.[12]

Human nature is seen as essentially good, since it is an expression of the Tao, nature in a larger sense.

> The Master Confucius said: Ch'ien and K'un are indeed the gate of Yi (Change)! Ch'ien is Yang and K'un is Yin. When Yin and Yang are united in their character, the weak and the strong attain their substance. In this way the products of Heaven and Earth

are given substance and the character of spiritual intelligence can be penetrated.[13]

The relative principles of Heaven (Yang, Tao, the creative) and Earth (Yin, De, virtue, character) unite with each other to form substance and spirit. The *I Ching* is the oldest book of China, the classic of classics. It has deeply influenced the whole of Chinese philosophy and culture, and even now it actively affects Chinese society and culture. The *I Ching* was written to help people conceptualize and perceive the rules of the environment, heaven, destiny, and the future, so that they might try their best to create and enjoy a better life. Everybody can use the *I Ching*. The students of the *I Ching* need to practice Yin and Yang, openness and balance. You might say this is very easy, but it's not. All people have their own *I Ching*: Yin and Yang, and all must learn to manage their own changes and find what is unchanging.

Traditional Chinese medicine is based on the classic of internal medicine, *Huangdi Nei Jing* (hereafter referred to as *Nei Jing*), which consists of two parts: *Su Wen* (*Plain Questions*) and *Ling Shu* (*Miraculous Pivot*, also known as *Canon of Acupuncture*). Although its authorship is ascribed to the Yellow Emperor, actually the work was a product of various unknown authors in the Warring States Period (475–221 B.C.), and it is based on the *I Ching*. *Nei Jing*, *I Ching*, and Yin Yang theory were formed during almost the same period, with Yin Yang as their common precept. We can say that if the *I Ching* is Yang, the *Nei Jing* is Yin. If the *Nei Jing* is a door to the treasure-house of Chinese medical classics, then the *I Ching* is its key. Sun Si-miao (581–682 A.D.), a prominent physician of Tang Dynasty and the author of the famous classic *Qian Jin Yao Fang* (*Prescriptions Worth a Thousand Gold*) (652 A.D.), a compilation of the medical achievements before the 7th century, said that "if you do not study *I Ching*, you cannot understand medicine at all."[14]

The following is a very important paragraph from the *Nei Jing*:

> The Yellow Emperor said: Yin and Yang are the way of Heaven and Earth, the great principle and outline of everything, the parents of change, the root and source of life and death, the palace of gods. Treatment of disease should be based upon the roots (of Yin and Yang).[15]

From this quotation, you can see that like the *I Ching*, the *Nei Jing* emphasizes that Yin and Yang are the basic principle of the entire universe. Yin and Yang are the sole root of both Chinese culture and Chinese medicine, and this principle has also been the starting point for many philosophical movements. Medicine is only one of a diverse range of topics covered in the *I Ching*. Because its basic principles are beyond words, they are expressed as signs or symbols which can be applied to any circumstances. Therefore, since the very early days of Chinese history, the Confucianists, Taoists, Military Strategists and Political Strategists (in the Warring States Period) have all used the *I Ching* as a theoretical basis for writings in many fields, including mathematics, science, government, the arts, physical exercise and meditation.

The system of thought of the *I Ching* not only formed the basis of China's native religion, Taoism, it also blended with other philosophies brought to China from abroad and, in turn, influenced cultures outside of China. In recent history, the Germans and related cultures have studied Chinese culture most deeply of all Westerners, one example being Richard Wilhelm's translation of the *I Ching*. The 18th century German philosopher and mathematician Gottfried Wilhelm Leibnitz developed a two-valued logic theory which was found to correspond to the binary arrangement of the sixty-four hexagrams of *I Ching*. The invention of the modern electronic computer, based on Leibnitz' binary numbers, can therefore be seen as a manifestation of the mathematical logic of *I Ching*. The connection between the *I Ching*, the remote classic, and computer science, the newest technology, is illustrated on the facing page.

| | | | | | | | | |
|---|---|---|---|---|---|---|---|---|
| 0 | | | ▬ ▬ | | | | | |
| 1 | | | ▬▬▬ | | | | | |

| Eight Trigrams | Kun | Gen | Kan | Sun | Zhen | Li | Dui | Qian |
|---|---|---|---|---|---|---|---|---|
| Decimal system | 0 | 1 | 2 | 3 | 4 | 5 | 6 | 7 |
| Binary system | 000 | 001 | 010 | 011 | 100 | 101 | 110 | 111 |

| Wuchi | Empty Ultimate | 0 |
|---|---|---|
| Taichi | Grand Ultimate | 1 |
| Liang Yi | Two Modes | $2 \times 1$ |
| Si Xiang | Four Forms | $2 \times 2$ |
| Ba Gua | Eight Trigrams | $2 \times 2 \times 2$ |
| 64 Gua | 64 Hexagrams | $2 \times 2 \times 2 \times 2 \times 2 \times 2$ |

Numbers and mathematics form the language of science. Just as mathematics allows scientific concepts to be expressed simply and clearly, the symbols Yin ▬ ▬ and Yang ▬▬▬ and the trigrams simplify and clarify philosophy and thinking. Western science is beginning to work with many of the ideas expressed in the *I Ching*. Space and time, particle and wave, (Yin and Yang), are now seen as relative rather than absolute and separate. The philosophy of the *I Ching* is found in modern physics (quantum mechanics): the basic rule of the Uncertainty Principle of Werner Karl Heisenberg (1901–1976) states that it is impossible to determine both the position and the speed of a particle simultaneously with any accuracy, since the act of measurement affects what is being measured. The *I Ching* can be viewed as a comprehensive compendium of the sciences, including cosmology, astronomy, geology, physics, physiology, philosophy, mathematics, computer science, and others, and it also includes spiritualism and divination.

Yin Yang and the Trigrams are also the symbols of spirit, and they represent the most important expression of the third-level culture. Just as modern science has probed the nature of the universe, enabling us to understand its mysteries, understanding the mysteries of *I Ching* will enable us to explore our inner universe and draw upon its resources. What may seem to be beyond apparent logic may ultimately be the true natural order of the universe.

# CHAPTER 4
# Confucius and Confucianism

To study a race or nation, we need to understand its nature, its culture, and its history. One way to do this is by finding and studying some individuals who best represent that culture. To understand Western culture, we might look at the life of Jesus and the writings about him; to understand India, we can study Sakyamuni Buddha; to understand China, we need to study its two great representatives, Confucius and Lao-tzu. Contemporary written accounts of both of them exist. They lived in a very special period, during which the world had many great people: Aristotle, Sakyamuni Buddha, Jesus, and others.

Confucius lived from 551 to 479 B.C. His major occupations were educator and government official. In the latter part of his life he became a wandering teacher; followed by his students, he would "preach to kings and vassal lords his doctrines of the functions of the ruler and the duties of the governed."[16] He spent his last years compiling notes on his teachings and editing the existing classics. The Chinese refer to their traditional literature as the "Si Shu Wu Jing," or "Four Books and Five Classics." Confucius contributed greatly to these texts.


Five Classics

*Shi Jing* (*The Book of Poetry*), a collection of 305 poems and folk songs dated from the 11th century B.C. to the 6th century B.C., probably first compiled in the early 6th century B.C. Its archaic language and intimate knowledge of Zhou customs mark it as genuinely old.

*Shu Jing* (*The Book of History*), a collection of records, speeches, and state papers dating possibly as far back as 2000 B.C., reflecting early and middle Zhou styles.

*I Ching* (*The Book of Change*).

*Li Ji* (*The Book of Rites*), rules for ceremonial etiquette on public and private occasions, documents and traditions of the Zhou Dynasty.

*Chun Qiu* (*Spring and Autumn Annals or Annals of Lu*), a chronicle of events in the State of Lu for the years 722–464 B.C.[17]

Four Books

*The Great Learning* (*Da Xue*), sayings of Confucius, giving his politico-moral philosophy for a ruler, collated by his disciples.

*The Doctrine of the Mean* (*Zhong Yong*), sayings of Confucius on the topic "The Human Mind in Itself and Its Expression According to the Will of Heaven" compiled by Tsu Ssu (Zu Si), grandson of Confucius, and others. It is the most important book of Confucianism.

*The Analects of Confucius* (*Lun Yu*), discourses of the Sage with his disciples, edited by them or collated by their immediate disciples.

*The Book of Mencius* (*The Meng Zi*) containing rules of righteous government, the qualities of a good ruler, notes on human nature, duty, etc., purporting to be the teachings of the Confucian commentator Mengzi (about 371–289 B.C.).[18]

In ancient times the Chinese said *The Great Learning* was the blueprint and the building process of a construction project, the *Doctrine of the Mean* was the foundation, the *Analects* and the *Book of Mencius* were the building materials of very high quality; but the building materials were scattered all over the ground, and it would require the hard work of architects and engineers before they could be sorted out and assembled into a building. We can compare constructing a building with educating a person. The materials can be assembled into a magnificent palace, a spacious and comfortable house, or a simple cottage. Most important is the foundation.

Confucius promoted moral behavior and tried to convince rulers to bring about improvements in the country. The title conferred upon him was "Teacher for all ages"; his works were the model for all people, and political factions made use of his teachings to strengthen their own rule. This, however, created conflicts between different groups which were for or against Confucius's political ideas.

Actually, there are two different components of Confucianism: the earlier Rujia (Confucian school of philosophy) and the later Kongjiao (Confucian religion). The Rujia represents a political-philosophical tradition which was extremely important in imperial times and is the element most directly connected with the doctrine of Confucius and Mengzi. The Kongjiao represents the state's efforts to meet the religious needs of the people within the framework of the Confucian tradition, an unsuccessful attempt which occurred in the late imperial period.[19] For some 2,000 years, Confucianism enjoyed almost unassailable prestige as the ideology of the imperial bureaucracy, an essential element of China's political unity. Regardless of how much a particular ruler might prefer Buddhism or Taoism, Confucianism had a practical importance in the affairs of government which could not be denied or neglected. Philosophical Confucianism was very successful as a political ideology, as well as being an impressive system of moral philosophy.[20]

Confucian theory is an easy way to bridge Eastern culture and Western science. Confucius's principles are recognized today throughout the world, and his sayings are often quoted by contemporary politicians. However, people who use Confucian philosophy need to understand it, and particularly its relationship to the *I Ching* theories. Relating Confucian philosophy to Taichi philosophy, we could compare Zhong Yong (the Golden Mean) to Yin Yang balance, and sincerity to the Taichi circle.

Studying both the *I Ching* and the *Zhong Yong* is like balancing Yin and Yang. The idea of the Golden Mean derives from *I Ching* philosophy. The following two illustrations show the connection between the Confucian Mean and Yin Yang balance as expressed in the *I Ching*.

The Mean is the center in the sense of keeping to the midway and not going to extremes or overindulging. The combination of Yin 1-3-7-9 and Yang 2-4-6-8 with 5 in the center is found in the ancient Chinese works *Gwei* [*Gui*] *Shu Tu* (*The Picture of*

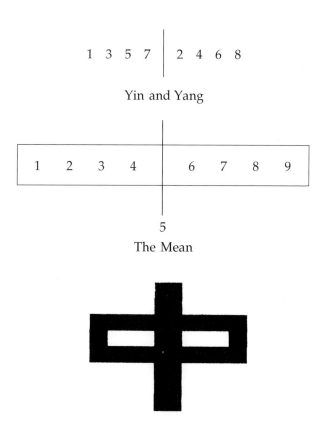

1  3  5  7  |  2  4  6  8

Yin and Yang

| 1 | 2 | 3 | 4 | | 6 | 7 | 8 | 9 |

5

The Mean

Chinese character for center

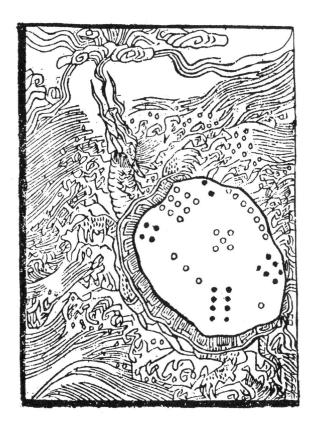

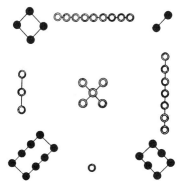

*the Wonder Turtle*), and *Luoh* [*Luo*] *Shu* (*The Book of River Luoh*).[21] The numerical marks on the turtle's back are symbolic language which represent the Mean and Yin Yang balance.

Besides **Zhong** (the Golden Mean), the term **Xing** (Hsing) defines another very important concept in Confucian philosophy. Xing is usually translated as nature, and can refer to temper, disposition, quality, property or characteristic, and in Buddhism to the true self. Another meaning of Xing is sex, and translating it as such gives us new insight into the classics. Regarding Xing, much was said in *The Doctrine of the Mean* about nature and character, but eating habits and sex were rarely mentioned. Sex is most basic to our nature, but the works of Confucius do not often address the subject. Five thousand years ago in China, sex was no doubt very open. Yin and Yang, the basic principle of *I Ching*, means female and male, woman and man. Only one side, only Yin or Yang, only man or woman, is not complete, not perfect. We need to combine and unite both Yin and Yang, female and male, woman and man.

Sex is very natural—it should not be a mysterious secret. If Confucius were alive today, perhaps he would talk openly about sex. Even in the Confucian classics we can find many positive viewpoints on sex, for example:

> Food and drink and the sexual relation between men and women compose the major human desires.[22]

> Eating food and having sex is the nature of human beings.[23]

Sex exists on the material level in humans as well as in animals. On this level, sex and food are basic and natural, and both are never completely satisfied. Food and sex can both be major fixations. You want to eat at a well-set table with flowers, music, proper lighting, good service, and so on, and a few hours later you need to eat again. If you depend on this kind of comfort you can never get enough. We need to develop and enjoy the higher culture, the third level culture, and practice the Doctrine of the Mean, not overdoing anything.

Comparing Xing (nature) with **Cheng** (sincerity) in Confucian thought, the notion of Cheng is prevalent. The universe is seen as one organism moved by the energy of sincerity.

> In *The Doctrine of The Mean* we find these interpretations of sincerity: "Sincerity is the way of heaven"; "Perfect sincerity is never static. Being never static makes things enduring. Being enduring makes things effective. Being effective makes things far-reaching and everlasting. Being far-reaching and everlasting makes things all-inclusive, and being all-inclusive makes things shine in brightness."

> This great energy comes from the self. It has the power to go into the heart of things and bring out knowledge, illuminating the darkness of ignorance. The more sincere one is, the brighter shines the light, and vice versa. Thus *The Doctrine of the Mean* says, "sincerity brings light, and light brings sincerity."

> Sincerity is energy, and energy manifests itself in the form of waves, such as light waves, sound waves, electric waves and electromagnetic waves. The waves can be converged. When light waves are converged in a single point, that point is called the focus and is the brightest spot. That is why we say "sincerity brings light."[24]

*The Doctrine of the Mean* says: "There are five enlightened moral orders in the world, and three virtues by which to practice them." The moral orders are relations governing interactions between ruler and subject, between one generation and the next, between spouses, between siblings, and between friends. The virtues are wisdom, benevolence and courage. And as Zhu Xi (Chu Hsi,

1130–1200 A.D.) says in his annotations, there is only one way to practice them: sincerity.

> The word sincerity contains several meanings; in the phrase "sincerity brings light," it means that without sincerity there is no wisdom; in "helping yourself as well as others" it means that sincerity and benevolence are one; in "perfect sincerity is never static," it means that through sincerity, courage can be brought out. The aggregate meaning of sincerity, however, is "to abide by the good, and persist to the end." "Only through sincerity can one fully bring out what is in oneself; only through sincerity can one go forward bravely, persisting from the beginning to the end; only through sincerity can one create, strive forward, and even make sacrifices."[25]

In studying the *Zhong Yong*, one finds that the way of heaven is called Xing, the straightforwardness or absence of hesitancy of character is called Tao, and cultivating the Tao is called education. Chapter 21 of the *Zhong Yong* says,

> By our nature, sincerity brings enlightenment. Through education, enlightenment brings sincerity. Given sincerity, there will be enlightenment, and given enlightenment, there will be sincerity.[26]

Studying and practice require sincerity and self-respect. To practice sincerity you need to devote yourself to something: Taichi Chuan, scientific research, etc. Students of Chinese medicine must have sincerity toward their own learning and achievements. That is why we say sincerity is the power and motivation behind a medical student. Sincerity is your key. In *The Doctrine of the Mean*, it is the motivation of everything, the source of life, the basis of human existence. It has been said that "with perfect sincerity, there is nothing that cannot be moved; without sincerity, nothing can be moved" and "where there is sincerity, even metals and rocks respond to its influence."

# CHAPTER 5
# Lao-tzu and Taoism

Laozi (Lao Tzu, or Lao-tzu) was used as the title of his book, *Lao Tzu* or *Tao Te Ching*, as well as the name of the writer. Lao-tzu's book is so important for China that we can even say that Chinese civilization and the Chinese character would have been utterly different if the book *Lao-tzu* had never been written. No one can hope to understand Chinese philosophy, religion, government, art, medicine—or even cooking—without a real appreciation of the profound philosophy taught in this little book. It is true that, while Confucianism emphasizes social order and an active life, Taoism concentrates on individual life, nature, and tranquility. This philosophy is embodied in a small classic of about 5,250 Chinese characters. No other Chinese classic of such small size has exercised so much influence. More commentaries have been written on it than on any other Chinese classic. About 350 are extant, besides some 350 that are lost or found only in fragment. There are also more English translations of it than of any other Chinese book—already over forty (in 1963).[27]

What is Tao?

There was something formless and perfect
before the universe was born.
It is serene. Empty.
Solitary. Unchanging.
Infinite. Eternally present.
It is the mother of the universe.
For lack of a better name, I call it the Tao.

It flows through all things,
inside and outside, and returns
to the origin of all things.
The Tao is great.
The universe is great.
Earth is great.
Man is great.
These are the four great powers.
Man follows the earth.
Earth follows the universe.
The universe follows the Tao.
The Tao follows only itself.[28]

We see here that the Tao is similar to the Taichi circle. Another poem from the *Tao Te Ching* expresses the *I Ching* concept of Taichi generating Yin and Yang, which interplay to create the changes of the universe:

The Tao gives birth to One.
One gives birth to Two.
Two gives birth to Three.
Three gives birth to all things.
All things have their backs to the female
and stand facing male.
When male and female combine,
all things achieve harmony.[29]

To understand Tao we need to understand Yin and Yang, and Three into One. As we read in the *I Ching* (The Appendix, I), "One Yin and One Yang constitute what is the Tao."[30] We cannot talk about 1 (Yin or Yang) by itself—we must talk about Yin and Yang together, which is 2. The invisible circle made by Yin and Yang is Taichi, or 3, which encompasses Yin and Yang, or 1 and 2. For example, to understand Heaven, we also need to talk about **Te**, Earth. According to traditional Chinese culture Heaven and Mankind are one, and celestial phenomena and the behavior of people are closely related. Where Heaven or Tao is Yang, Earth or

| Tao | Ren | Te |
|---|---|---|
| heaven | people | earth |
| way | benevolence | virtue |
| spiritual | societal | material |
| invisible | visible | visible |
| hard to control | can be controlled | can be controlled |
| absolute | relative | relative |

Te is Yin. Between Heaven and Earth is the Confucian principle of **Ren**, humanity or compassion.

> There is a path lying between man and man. That path is the way [tao], and how to walk along the path is te (the power which realizes the moral law). Says Chu Hsi, "To practice the moral way in accordance with the dictates of your heart, that is te."[31]

Lao-tzu was against political corruption and believed in an ideal society devoted to selflessness, and to a mystical union with the One. He was in favor of recovering the original aspect of the Chinese culture and transmitting it to posterity. Because Confucius talked about government and politics, his doctrines were used by emperors to control people, so he became controversial. With Lao-tzu everything was nature; he created a work of art and a universal Taichi philosophy of Three into One (see illustration on the next page). In the Confucian Doctrine of the Mean, the two ends define the center; with Lao-tzu there is a third, unseen point. In Mainland China, especially during the so-called "Cultural Revolution," the Communists destroyed the works of Confucius, but not those of Lao-tzu. Even though in his later days Lao-tzu could not escape economics, politics and religion, he retreated to the mountains rather than get involved in the world, and so his mind is still with us. There is a legend that during their lifetimes, Confucius visited Lao-tzu and tried to get answers to philosophical questions from him. Taoism, like Confucianism, has both a philosophical and a religious

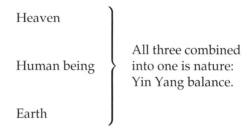

Heaven

Human being          All three combined
                     into one is nature:
                     Yin Yang balance.

Earth

tradition. Although philosophical Taoism flourished early, in the 5th century B.C., Taoism as a religion did not develop until the 1st century A.D.[32] Lao-tzu emphasizes Nature. Many of the techniques of self-cultivation such as Taichi Chuan, Chi Kung (Qi Gong), and meditation were derived from the teachings of Lao-tzu. Taichi Chuan is often regarded as a Taoist system of exercise for the prolongation of life and eternal youth, and Lao-tzu is credited as its father. Here is an account of the origins and historical development of the Yang School of Taichi Chuan:

> The principles of Taichi Chuan originated with Lao-tzu, who said, "Concentrate your Chi [Qi] on becoming supple." It was during the Tang Dynasty... however, that two men, Xu Xuanping (Hsu Hsuan-ping) and Li Daozhi (Li Tao-Tzu, or Li Tao-Shan, who was called the master of Wudang), transformed Lao-tzu's abstract ideas into a particular form. They called it "chang quan" (the continuous blow) to emphasize its inexhaustible, never-ending character.
>
> Xu was a native of Shi District in Huizhou, Anhui Province. He later retreated to Ziyang Mountain in Shanxi Province. Li's ancestral home was in Anhui. He retreated to Nanyan Temple on Wudang Mountain in Hubei Province and taught Zhang Sanfeng (Chang San-Feng, 1279–1386 A.D.), patriarch of the Wudang School, legendary founder of Taichi Quan

and author of *The Sanfeng Taichi Classic*. Zhang was from Liaodong in Yizhou in Liaoning Province.

Patriarch Zhang taught Wang Zhongyue (or Wang Zhong, Wang Tsung), who lived during the Ming Dynasty (1368–1644 A.D.). Wang became famous for his refined skill. He also changed the name "chang quan" to Taichi Chuan and wrote *The Theory of Taichi Quan*. Wang taught Chen Zhoutong (Chen Chow-tung) from Wenzhou, Zhejiang Province. Chen taught Zhang Songxi (Chang Sung Chi) of Yin District in Zhejiang Province. Zhang taught Ye Jimei (Yeh Chi-Mei). Ye taught Shan Sinan. Shan taught Wang Zhengnan of the Qing (Ch'ing) Dynasty (1644–1911 A.D.). Zhengnan then taught Yang Luchan from Hebei Province. Yang Luchan (Yang Lu Ch'an, 1799–1872 A.D.) was the originator of the currently flourishing Yang-style (Yang Family Hidden Tradition) Taichi Quan. He taught his second son Banhou (Yang Pan-Hou, 1837–1892), and his third son Jianhou (Yang Chien-Hou, 1839–1917) and others. This school was taught by Banhou to Wanchun, Quanyou, Leshan, and others, and by Jianhou to Chengfu, who taught Zhang Qinlin and others.

Zhang Qinlin was a native of Xingtai County in Hebei and lived in Taiyuan City in Shanxi Province. He taught Cheng Manching, Wang Sanzhi, and Li Yunlung of Hebei; and Hu Yaozhen, Liu Zhiliang, Su Qigeng and Wang Yen-nien of Shanxi Province.[33]

Wang Yen-nien was my teacher, and now I am an overseas teacher of the Yang-style Taichi Chuan and the Taichi Tao Tradition. This style of Taichi emphasizes not only Yin Yang balance, but also the integration of mind, breath and action, Three into One.

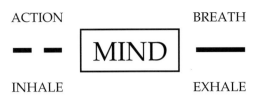

# CHAPTER 6
# Buddhism and Chinese Culture

Buddhism is not a native religion in China. It was introduced into China from India.

> Out of the life-experience and teaching of high-born Prince Siddhartha Gautama of the Sakya clan in the kingdom of Magadha, who lived from 560 or 550 to 477 B.C., sprang the religious philosophy we know as Buddhism.[34]

> Reduced to its simplest form, the teaching of Buddha has been set forth traditionally in the "Four Noble Truths," ... that life is full of suffering; suffering is caused by passionate desires, lusts, cravings; only as these are obliterated will suffering cease; such eradication of desire may be accomplished only by following the Eightfold Path of earnest endeavor.[35]

In the centuries after the life of Sakyamuni Buddha, Buddhism in India developed into many schools with differences in doctrine and practice, generally influenced by Hindu philosophy. These are divided into two major branches. Hinayana Buddhism, also known as the Theravada (conservative) school or the Lesser vehicle, was predominant in the south of India, while Mahayana Buddhism (Sarvastivada or liberal school) developed in the north of India.

**39**

It was Mahayana Buddhism that spread to China, beginning to develop in the middle of the second century. By the first quarter of the third century, there were two Buddhist movements of thought in China: dhyana (concentration) and prajna (wisdom).

> The objective of dhyana was so to meditate and to achieve calmness of mind as to remove ignorance and delusions, while that of prajna was to gain the wisdom that things possess no self-nature (svabhava).[36]

Sakyamuni Buddha is said to have spent 22 of his 49 years of teaching expounding the prajna SutraHeart Sutra. The prajna Sutra contains the essence of the deepest Buddhist teachings. Its special characteristics are explained in Jia Ming Guan (The View of Supposition). Its basic statement affirms that mankind has the absolute and full capacity for knowing. One's degree of acknowledgement and attitude determine whether one can utilize this ability to fully recognize all the truth of the universe and human life. The 260-word Heart Sutra is the essence of the prajna Sutra. If you read the Heart Sutra and can realize the deep meaning contained in it, you will have found the entrance to Buddhism.

The following is an English translation of the Heart Sutra (Prajnaparamitahridaya);[37]

### The Heart Sutra

> When the Bodhisattva Avalokitesvara was engaged in the practice of the deep Prajnaparamita, he perceived that there are the five Skandhas; and these he saw in their self-nature to be empty.
>
> O Sariputra, form is here emptiness, emptiness does not differ from form, form does not differ from emptiness; that which is form is emptiness, that which is emptiness is form. The same can be said of sensation, thought, conception, and consciousness.
>
> O Sariputra, all things here are characterized with emptiness: they are not born, they are not annihi-

lated; they are not tainted, they are not immaculate; they do not increase, they do not decrease.

Therefore, O Sariputra, in emptiness there is no form, no sensation, no thought, no conception, no consciousness; no eye, ear, nose, tongue, body, mind; no form, sound, color, taste, touch, objects; no sight-organ element, and so forth, until we come to: no mind-consciousness element. There is no ignorance, no extinction of ignorance, and so forth, until we come to: there is no decay and death, no extinction of decay and death. There is no suffering, no origination of suffering, no stopping of suffering, no path. There is no knowledge, no attainment, no realization, because there is no attainment. In the mind of the Bodhisattva who dwells depending on the Prajna-paramita (perfection of wisdom) there are no obstacles; and, foregoing the perverted views, he reaches final Nirvana. All the Buddhas of the past, present, and future, depending on the Prajnaparamita, attain to the highest perfect enlightenment.

Therefore, one ought to know that the Prajna-paramita is the great Mantram, the Mantram of great wisdom, the highest Mantram, the peerless Mantram, which is capable of allaying all suffering; it is truth because it is not falsehood: this is the Mantram proclaimed in the Prajnaparamita. It runs: "Gate, gate, paragate, parasamgate, bodhi, svaha!" (O Bodhi, gone, gone, gone to the other shore, landed at the other shore, Svaha!)[38]

A Bodhisattva is an enlightened being who has postponed escape from the world of birth and death in order to help others. Prajnaparamita is wisdom which has gone beyond everything earthly yet has left none of it behind. The Skandas, heaps, or Five Elements are: form, feeling (sense-perception), thought (ideation), conception (conformation), and consciousness. Emptiness in Mahayana Buddhism means absolute, with no limiting qualities. It denotes liberation from the world around us and absence of any kind of relative self. (These explanations of terms in the Heart Sutra are based on opinions in Conze.[39] The following illustration contains the text of the Heart Sutra.[40])

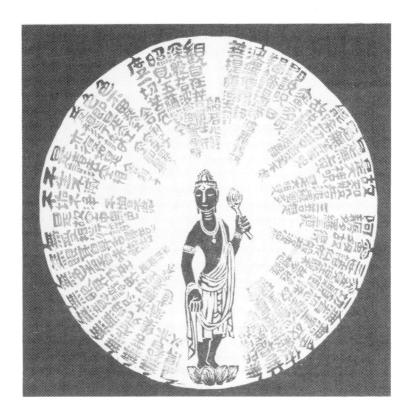

Chinese Buddhism continued to develop into schools based upon the Indian Buddhist tradition, but Buddhist thought was translated in terms of existing Chinese philosophy. Many sects developed in China after the 4th century. The Pure Land School, founded by a Taoist monk in the 4th century, became a devotional religious philosophy of salvation by faith. The Madhyamika School was brought to China in the same period through a Tibetan who translated many works and transmitted them to Taoist pupils. In the following century, the Tiantai School emphasized harmony among the sects and universal salvation through concentration and insight.[41]

Tang Xuan Zhuang (Hsuan-tsang) was a monk of the Pure Land School who had studied all the Chinese texts on Buddhism and was determined to find answers to his questions about the doctrines. Tang is said to have travelled in about 633 A.D. to the Buddhist University of Nalanda in northern India, becoming the first Chinese scholar to study in a foreign country. He brought with him Lao-tzu's *Tao Te Ching*, which he translated into Sanskrit. When he returned to China, Tang was given imperial patronage to translate Buddhist literature into Chinese.

The essence of Chinese Buddhism is to differentiate Jia Ming (the Superficial Name) from Shi Xiang (the Real Appearance), which are termed Yin and Yang. The highest concept in Buddhism is explained by Taichi (the Great Ultimate). The *I Ching* and the *Tao Te Ching* provide the basis for Chinese people to understand the Heart Sutra and other Buddhist classics. Looking into the inner core, we can find correlations among Taoism, Confucianism, and Buddhism:

| Taoism | Yin | Yang | Taichi (Great Ultimate) |
|---|---|---|---|
| Confucianism | benevolence | love | Cheng (Sincerity) |
| Buddhism | form | emptiness | prajna (Perfect Wisdom) |

Chanting the Heart Sutra with sincerity can help people to open. We are only restricted by our own hangups. Hangup is a very close translation of the Chinese word Zhizhou (or Zhimibuwu). A hangup refers to anything which a person allows to enmesh his or her mind in petty detail, preventing it from experiencing the larger meaning beyond. Although it originated as a Buddhist term, we can also understand it in terms of Yin Yang theory. While a hangup is Yin and closed, its opposite, open-mindedness, is Yang and open. Form and emptiness are like Yin and Yang, open mind is like Taichi.

# CHAPTER 7
# Zen and Chinese Culture

The mixture of Buddhism with Taoism in China developed into **Chan Xue**, known in the West as Zen Buddhism. The word "Xue," like the suffix -ology, means study. The word Zen (Chan) comes from the Sanskrit word for meditation, Dhyana, but actually the Zen principles differ from Indian Dhyana Buddhism to the extent that the former are related to Yin Yang theory. Zen Buddhism later spread to Japan, and then to America. The Zen Movement has been described by Dr. Daisetz Teitaro Suzuki as a movement in which "the Chinese mind completely asserted itself, in a sense, in opposition to the Indian mind. Zen could not rise and flourish in any other land or among any other people."[42]

Zen may therefore be regarded as the fullest development of Taoism by wedding it to the congenial Buddhist insights and the powerful Buddhist impulse of apostolic zeal. If Buddhism is the father, Taoism is the mother of this prodigious child. But there can be no denying that the child looks more like the mother than the father.[43]

Literally, the name of the school should be Meditation, for the Sanskrit Dhyana, pronounced in Chinese "ch'an" and in Japanese "zen," means that. But meditation changed its character in China almost from the very inception of Buddhism, although the typically Indian form of sitting in meditation and concentrating one's mind to the point of ignoring the external world has continued in Chinese Buddhist schools. When Buddhism first came to China, it was mixed up with the Yellow Emperor-Lao Tzu cult. As a result, meditation was not understood in the Indian sense of concentration but in the Taoist sense of conserving vital energy, breathing, reducing desire, preserving nature, and so forth. This was the meditation taught by early Buddhist Masters like An Shih-kao (An Shigao, c. A.D. 150), Kumarajiva (344–413 A.D.), Tao-an (312–385), and Hui-yuan (334–416). In the end, meditation meant neither sitting in meditation nor mental concentration, but simply the direct enlightenment of the mind.[44]

... There can be no greater difference in meaning between two terms than the Indian "Dhyana" and the Chinese "Ch'an." Dhyana signifies a concentrated and methodical meditation, while Zen, as the founding fathers of the Chinese School understood it, has for its essence a sudden flash of insight into Reality, or a direct intuitive perception of the Self-nature.[45]

In its initial form in Indian Dhyana, the approach is to lead believers in gradually, emphasizing harmony of mind, breath, and the whole body. The goal is to get into a state of complete cessation of thought so that the heart is in complete tranquility and the mind is able to concentrate on the unity of the body and the outside environment. Zen in China absorbed this original meaning, but its spirit changed when it blended with the existing Chinese culture. In Zen the emphasis is on sudden realization of truth, or an awakening in a flash. This will enable a person to go directly into the lands of Rulai (the title for Sakyamuni Buddha), arrive at absolute emptiness, and immerse naturally in the magical effect: Wisdom. The Indian Dhyana placed its emphasis on gradualism, in practicing Buddhist conduct. Although the two are in different domains, neither can be discarded, because they are relevant to each other and supplement each other. Zen closely associates Dhyana with daily life (sitting, lying, walking) and does not limit itself to the time of meditation, striving for the ideal situation where Zen is life and life is Zen.

The evolution of Zen begins with Ta-Mo (Damo, Bodhidharma), the twenty-eighth Indian Patriarch of the Mahayana school, who arrived in Canton in the late 5th or early 6th century and became the first Patriarch of the Zen school. Ta-Mo is said to have sat facing a wall in the Shao Lin Monastery, exemplifying his doctrine of deep contemplation. It was with the teaching of Hung-jen (Hongren) in the 7th century that Chinese Buddhism began to take on the character of what we know as Zen today. Hung-jen emphasized the mind rather than an external Ultimate Reality as its central focus. His disciples, Shen-hsiu (Shenxiu) and Hui-Neng, continued his teaching, but diverged from each other in stressing gradual enlightenment of the mind versus sudden enlightenment.

Shenxiu:

The body is the tree of Puti.
The mind is the stand of a bright mirror.
Wipe it constantly and with ever-watchful diligence,
To keep it uncontaminated by the worldly dust.[46]

Hui-Neng:

Puti is no tree,
Nor is the Bright Mirror a stand.
Since it is not a thing at all,
Where could it be contaminated by dust?[47]

Hui-Neng's sudden enlightenment is the basic principle of Chinese Zen. The following is an outline of the four interdependent points in Hui-Neng's teaching.

First, Dharma, or Reality and Truth, can only be transmitted from mind to mind. A Zen master cannot infuse his own insights

into the mind of another but can be present like a midwife helping at a birth. Second, we should not be dependent on words
and writings or be attached to expounding the scriptures. Third,
pointing directly at the mind is a step toward understanding the
self-nature. The mind of our thoughts is not the real mind, since
the real mind is that which is thinking, not that which is thought
about. In speaking of the mind we are at best pointing to the
pointing. There must be a leap beyond the superficial level of
the words of our thoughts, a breakthrough to the higher level of
Reality. The mind is a dynamic process which must go on in a
never-ending flow; like a river it is sometimes pure and sometimes muddy. "No-thought" means letting the mind function
actively and freely in all things without attachment to anything.
Fourth, to perceive the self-nature is to attain Buddhahood. Our
original nature is Buddha. The self-nature is identical with the
non-dual Real, which is beyond space and time and above all
attributes that human language can offer.[48]

Zen is philosophically consistent with Tao and the *Tao Te Ching*.
Hui-Neng stated that:

> Light and darkness are two different things in the
> eyes of the ordinary people. But the wise and under-
> standing ones possess a penetrating insight that there
> can be no duality in the self-nature. The Non-dual
> nature is the Real Nature. The Real Nature does not
> decrease in the fool nor increase in the sage; it is un-
> perturbed in the midst of trials, nor does it stay still
> in the depth of meditation and samadhi; it is nei-
> ther impermanent nor permanent; it neither comes
> nor goes; it is neither in the middle, nor in the inte-
> rior, nor in the exterior; it is not born and does not
> die; both its essence and its manifestations are in the
> absolute state of suchness. Eternal and unchanging,
> we call it the "Tao."[49]

This viewpoint is similar to the first chapter of the *Tao Te Ching*:

> The tao that can be told
> is not the eternal Tao.
> The name that can be named
> is not the eternal Name.
> The unnameable is the origin of Heaven and Earth;
> Naming is the creation
> of all particular things.
> By the eternity of unknown existence
> comprehend the common essence of things;
> By the eternity of Existence
> observe the apparent differences.
> These two came from the same origin—the unknown
> but with different names.
> They all are called the "profoundness" [**Hsuan**]
> Profoundly and profoundly it is the entrance
> from which come all wonders.[50]

The Tao in both Lao-tzu and Hui-Neng is eternal and unchangeable. The concepts of **Xin** (mind, heart) in Buddhism and **Wu** (enlightenment) in Zen are philosophically similar to the concept of Cheng (sincerity) in Confucianism.

> Hui-Neng's philosophy is as transcendental as that of Lao-tzu and Chuang Tzu; but at the same time it is as man-centered as that of Confucius and Mencius.[51]

Hui-Neng pointed out that:

> The Bodhi or Wisdom, which constitutes our self-nature, is pure from the beginning. We need only use our mind to perceive it directly to attain Buddhahood.[52]

This can be compared to the Confucian sayings cited earlier, "Sincerity brings light," which means that without sincerity there is no wisdom, and to "Sincerity is the way of heaven," which means that only sincerity can bring one to openness, just as only one's mind can bring one to attain Buddhahood.

> Hui-Neng, in his last instruction to his disciples, enumerated no less than thirty-six pairs of opposites. "... If you know the proper way of using these pairs of opposites, you will be able to go freely in and out through the scriptural Dharmas, steering clear of the two extremes by letting the self-nature stir and function spontaneously."[53]

This shows the characteristically Chinese application of Yin Yang theory to Buddhist philosophy. The purpose of awakening is to transform one's worries and attain **Bhodi** or Puti (true awakening, enlightenment). Hui-Neng said, "If good at acquiring knowledge, a mortal becomes Buddha, and worries will be like Puti. With the first thought you are lost, you're a mortal. With the second thought you awaken, you're Buddha. Previous thoughts, enclosed in the environment, become worries. Later thoughts, away from the environment, are Puti." Worries and Puti are two sides of the same thing, and the crucial factor is whether or not the awakening takes place at the split second. If awakening takes place, there will be no rigidity, no stubbornness, no inflexibility; then Puti heart will appear. If awakening does not take place, the mind is closed; a large number of worries will follow.

# CHAPTER 8
# Christianity and Chinese Culture

Christianity was introduced into China during the Tang Dynasty as early as 635 A.D., when Christian Nestorian missionaries from Syria arrived in Chang-an (now Xi'an), the capital of Tang Empire. Christianity was known in the form of "Jing Jiao" (Nestorianism) in ancient China. By the time it, as well as Buddhism, was forbidden in the Chinese Empire in 845 A.D., "Jing Jiao" already had more than 100 churches and more than 2,000 clergymen. In the Yuan Dynasty (Mongol, 1271–1368 A.D.), Catholics and Nestorians came to China again. At this time, the faith was called "Shizi (Cross) Jiao." It disappeared again with the fall of Yuan Dynasty.[54]

The rediscovery of China by Portuguese traders renewed the missionary interest of the Roman Catholic Church. Francis Xavier, who in 1549 introduced Catholicism to Japan, was the first zealot in the new campaign to convert the Chinese. Xavier, however died off the coast of Kwangtung (1552), thwarted in his ambition to carry Roman Catholicism to China. Xavier was followed by Matteo Ricci (in Chinese Li Ma Dou), an Italian Jesuit who reached Macao in 1582. The religious propaganda of Ricci, his associates, and successors, based on their appeal to the scientific and scholarly interests of Chinese officialdom, met with notable success. A century after Ricci's arrival at Canton, the K'ang-hsi emperor granted freedom of worship to the Roman churches throughout the empire. The official favors, however, did not exempt the missionaries from persecution. In 1616 and again in 1664 some of the Jesuits were expelled from Peking and forced to return to Canton or Macao.[55]

In the 19th century, coincident with the opening of China and Japan, Protestant Christendom became active in the field of foreign missions. In 1805 the London Missionary Society sent Robert Morrison to China. The American Bible Society also entered the field. During the first year of its work in China (1822), the Society distributed 500 copies of the New Testament. Eighty years later it was giving away more than half a million copies, including an elegantly bound edition to the Empress Dowager on her sixtieth birthday. After 1830, American Protestantism was represented in China by an expanding group of churches and missionary societies.[56]

Christianity has already become a part of the Chinese culture. The following is a very good example:

> T'ai-p'ing-T'ian-Kuo was a great peasant rebellion in Ching Dynasty, from 1851 to 1864, lasting as long as 14 years. It was not a replica of a familiar pattern, for the Taipings were not merely peasant rebels, but social and cultural revolutionaries as well. Hung Hsiu-ch'uan (1814–64), the leader of the Taipings, was a country intellectual. During visits to Canton to study for and participate in the examinations, he came into contact with Protestant missionary tracts, and, briefly, with missionaries themselves. Through some complex psychological process, he had a series of visionary experiences and came to believe that he was the younger brother of Jesus Christ, whose mission on earth was to extirpate the evils that infested Chinese society and to establish a Heavenly Kingdom in China. The quasi-Christian "Society of God Worshippers" which Hung and a friend organized in 1846–47 soon came into conflict with the local gen-

try, and eventually with the government. By 1850 he and his followers were in open revolt against the Manchu Dynasty. The rebellion spread rapidly over southeastern China, and then moved northward. In 1853 Nanking was captured and made the capital of the T'ai-P'ing-T'ian-Kuo, or Heavenly Kingdom of Great Peace. Here, Hung ruled as T'ien Wang (Heavenly King) until the city fell to Ch'ing armies in 1864. This rebellion under the banner of God and Christianity, at one time or another, penetrated sixteen of the eighteen provinces of China proper.[57] In this new theocracy God was the Heavenly Father; Christ, the Divine Elder Brother; and the T'ai-P'ing Wang (Hung himself) the Divine Younger Brother. The Christian factor in the movement was, in the main, the first five books of the Old Testament.[58]

Here is one of the songs of Taipings:

On Reverence for God

Let the true Spirit, the Great God,
Be honored and adored by all nations;
Let the many men and women of the world,
Morning and evening worship him alike.
Above and below, look where you may,
All things are imbued with God's favor.
At the beginning, in six days,
All things were created, perfect and complete.[59]

Like Buddhism, at its nucleus Christianity is compatible with traditional Chinese ideology, including Taoism and Confucianism. One interesting point to note is that Tao is God, according to the Chinese, who translate Gospel John 1:1 as "In the beginning was the Tao, and the Tao was with God, and the Tao was God."[60] In the English translation of the Bible, the Word is God. And according to the original Greek version of the Bible, Logos is God. The word Logos generally connotes life, light, creation, power, wisdom, love, healing, spirit, force, knowledge, rationality, logic, reality, and method. The Chinese word Tao has the same connotations. That is why the word Tao was used in the Chinese Biblical translation.[61] It was mentioned above that sincerity is a basic principle of Chinese culture. The concept of sincerity originated from the *I Ching*:[62]

> The Master (Confucius) said:—"There he is, with the dragon's powers, and occupying exactly the central place. He is sincere (even) in his ordinary words, and earnest in his ordinary conduct. Guarding against depravity, he preserves his sincerity."[63]

> The Master (Confucius) said:—"The superior man advances in virtue, and cultivates all the sphere of his duty. His real-heartedness and good faith are the ways by which he advances in virtue. His attention to his words and establishing his sincerity are the way by which he occupies his sphere."[64]

As we can see, Confucius is said to have first stated the principle of sincerity in the *I Ching*. Certainly, as we cited in Chapter 4, in *Zhong Yong* (*The Doctrine of the Mean*) the principle of sincerity was explored very clearly, deeply, and broadly. It is very important to understand that what is attributed to sincerity in *Zong Yong* is very similar to what is attributed to God in the Bible:[65]

### Zhong Yong and the New Testament

| | |
|---|---|
| Sincerity is the way of Heaven. The attainment of sincerity is men. <br> Zhong Yong 20–14 (p. 88)[66] | Jesus said to him: I am the way, and the truth, and the way of life. <br> John 14:6[67] |

But given the sincerity, and there shall be the intelligence and wisdom; given the intelligence, and there shall be the sincerity.
21:2 (p. 90)

O, the depth of the riches and wisdom and knowledge of God!
Romans 11:33

It is characteristic of the perfect sincerity to be able to foreknow.
24:1 (p. 95)

But the wisdom from above is first pure, then peaceful, gentle, open to reason, full of mercy and fruits, without uncertainty or insincerity.
James 3:17

Sincerity is the end and beginning of things; without sincerity there would be nothing.
25:2 (p. 96)

He (Tao) was in the beginning with God:  all things were made through him, and without him was not anything made that was made.
John 1:2-3

He who attains to sincerity is he who chooses what is good, and firmly holds it fast.
20:18 (p. 88)

But the Lord is faithful; he will strengthen you and guard you from evil.
2 Thessalonians 3:3

It is only he who possessed the perfect sinceritiy that can exist under heaven, who can transform.
23:3 (p. 94)

For with God nothing will be impossible.
Luke 137

It is only the individual possessed of the perfect sincerity that can exist under heaven, who can adjust the great invariable relations of mankind,

And you have come to fullness of life in him, who is the head of all rule and authority.
Colossians 2:10 (p. 574)

establish the great fundamental virtues of humanity, and
know the transforming and
nurturing operations of Heaven and Earth—shall this individual have any being or anything beyond himself on which
he depends?
32:1 (pp. 114–115)

These are just a few examples; there are many other scriptures showing correspondence between the concepts of God and Perfect Sincerity. We can see Yin and Yang in the Old Testament as well; for example, Noah's ark carried male and female pairs of animals.

There are many parallels between Christian ideas and the Taichi theory. Adam and Eve, Heaven and Hell, God and Satan, Death and Resurrection are all relative pairs, or Yin and Yang. The absolute is faith, belief or sincerity. In the idea of the Trinity, we can see Yin and Yang and the intangible Taichi absolute. Yin and Yang are just two; there has to be a transcending third aspect to balance them. True prayer requires sincerity. Faith and Sincerity is a way to teach oneself under the guidance of God.

It is very important to point out that Cheng (sincerity) and Xin (faith) are identical. Confucius, Lao-tzu and Jesus all ask people to be sincere and faithful to their belief. Taoism, Confucianism, and Christianity have the same goal—guiding people to learn and follow the Tao (Way). Whatever your belief, having faith as the third point allows you to balance good and evil, Yin and Yang.

Christianity impacted on China very much in another important field—medicine. The Roman Catholic church initiated missionary activity in China, with Matteo Ricci as one of the first missionaries in this wave, followed by Nicholaus Longobardi, Alphoso Vagnoni, and Francisco Sambiaso. They, the first to introduce European scientific knowledge and medicine into China, translated many books on science and medicine into Chinese. The Protestant church did not send its emissaries to China until the Ch'ing (Manchu) Dynasty (1644–1911). These included men with medical training who did much to introduce Western medicine into China in the 19th century. Their activities usually began in Hong Kong, Macao and Canton, thereafter gradually extending to the interior. Some of the early medical practitioners included: Alexander Pearson (arrived in China in 1805), Thomas Richardson Colledge (1827), Peter Parker (1834), William Lockhart and Benjamin Hobson (1839), and John Kerr from Glasgow, Scotland (1854). They established hospitals and medical schools in China and translated Western medical books into Chinese. Dr. John Kerr published the first Chinese journal of Western medicine, *Xiyi Xinbao* (*New Journal of Western Medicine*), in 1881, published by the Po T'si Hospital in Canton.[68] The next chapter looks at Western medicine from the perspective of traditional Chinese medicine.

# CHAPTER 9
# Western Medicine vis-a-vis Chinese Medicine

Wherever there are people, there is medicine. Human beings are one, and our bodies are basically the same whether from the West or the East. Traditional Chinese medicine and Western medicine study and treat the same human being. As long as we can cure people, it doesn't matter what kind of medicine we use.

In their beginnings, Eastern and Western medical ideas were almost the same: both saw the body in terms of two poles and four or five elements. In many of the deepest basic principles, such as homeostasis, there is no difference between the two medical traditions. Yet like the major rivers where civilizations originally developed, the path of culture flows and changes. This has led to cultural differences with strong impact on medicine. It is these differences in cultural, philosophical, and historical background which have made Western and Chinese medicine diverge. When Western medicine was introduced into China, the Chinese people welcomed it, and there has been a tendency to integrate Western medicine with traditional Chinese medicine. There is a Chinese saying, "Have the whole world in mind. Project a long-term cultural exchange between the human cultures." One must therefore understand Western medicine in order to fully understand Chinese medicine, particularly those aspects in which the two are parallel.[69]

## Medicine Before the Greeks

The beginnings of medicine are lost in antiquity. The history of Western medicine begins with the Greeks, but the art of healing had been practiced long before. It seems clear that each of the great civilizations that preceded or were contemporaneous with the Greeks had developed some form of the healing of wounds and the treatment of disease. The most famous ones were Chinese medicine along the Yellow River, Indian medicine along the Ganges River, and Egyptian medicine along the Nile River.

## Greek Medicine: Hippocrates and the Hippocratic Oath

In the third century B.C., Empedocles put forward the idea that the body was composed of equal parts of earth, air, fire, and water. Good health resulted from a correct balance of these elements. The elements, or humors as they were called, came to be equated with various body substances and dispositions. Thus the earth was equivalent to black bile (melanchole), and when dominant gave the individual a sad nature. The air was yellow bile (chole) and in excess led to a bad-tempered choleric personality. Fire was like the blood (sanguis) and produced a happy disposition, and water was phlegm (pituita) and made for a cold nature. These ideas, which were incorporated in the writings of the Hippocratic school, are similar to the Yin Yang and Five Elements theories of Chinese medicine. Although these conceptions have been discarded from Western scientific thought, they linger in the English language: we all know what is meant by a sanguine or a phlegmatic temperament, a bilious or a melancholy disposition.

The Greek physician Hippocrates (460–370 B.C.) is recognized as the father of Western medicine. He believed that people could find the laws of nature by studying facts and reasoning from them.  He placed medicine on a scientific basis through the practice of bedside observation of disease, which today is known as the experimental method.  By applying logic and reason to medicine, Hippocrates made the practice of medicine more workable.  He also showed that disease had only natural causes and took treatment of disease out of the hands of religion.  He treated his patients with proper diet, fresh air, change in climate, and attention to habits and living conditions.  He objected to the use of strong drugs without careful testing of their curative values.  His favorite diet for sick people was a barley gruel, and his favorite medicine was honey.  He said, "The drink to be employed should there be any pain is vinegar and honey.  If there be great thirst, give water and honey."  He also encouraged exercise and massage.  Like Chinese physicians, he believed that "Our natures are the physicians of our diseases."

A large number of medical works, extending over several centuries, were put together and became known as the Hippocratic collection.  It is in these writings that we find the famous Hippocratic Oath which lays down ethical standards for the practitioner.  The Hippocratic Oath, in its present form, may be of a later date than Hippocrates; and parts of it may be from an earlier time.  It reflects the ethics of the Hippocratic physicians.  It gave the medical profession a sense of duty to mankind which it has never lost, and many graduating medical students still take the oath with sincerity.  It includes the rules for the relationship between doctor and patients, and between doctors.

### HIPPOCRATIC OATH

"I swear by Apollo the physician, by Aesculapius, Hygeia, and Panacea, and I take to witness all the gods, all the goddesses to keep according to my ability and my judgement the following Oath:

To consider dear to me as my parents him who taught me this art; to live in common with him and if necessary to share my goods with him; to look upon

his children as my own brothers, to teach them this
art if they so desire without fee or written promise;
to impart to my sons and the sons of the master who
taught me and the disciples who have enrolled themselves and have agreed to the rules of the profession,
but to these alone, the precepts and the instruction.
I will prescribe regimen for the good of my patients
according to my ability and my judgement and never
do harm to anyone. To please no one will I prescribe
a deadly drug, nor give advice which may cause his
death. Nor will I give a woman a pessary to procure
abortion. But I will preserve the purity of my life and
my art. I will not cut for stone, even for patients in
whom the disease is manifest; I will leave this operation to be performed by practitioners (specialist in
this art). In every house where I come I will enter
only for the good of my patients, keeping myself far
from all intentional ill-doing and all seduction, and
especially from the pleasure of love with women or
with men, be they free or slaves. All that may come
to my knowledge in the exercise of my profession or
outside of my profession or in daily commerce with
men, which ought not to be spread abroad, I will
keep secret and will never reveal. If I keep this oath
faithfully, may I enjoy my life and practice my art,
respected by all men and in all times; but if I swerve
from it or violate it, may the reverse be my lot."[70]

The medical ethics of traditional Chinese medicine are similar
to those of Western medicine. Important principles of Chinese
medical ethics are found in the *Nei Jing* (the classic text of Chinese
medicine discussed in Chapter 3), approximately contemporary
with Hippocrates.

To make diagnosis without an adequate knowledge of Yin and Yang as well as upstream and down-
stream movements is the first fault on the part of

physician (due to inattentiveness). To quit in the middle of receiving instructions from teachers, to learn medical skills from phony schools of thought, to advertise one's medical skills falsely, to apply stone-needles indiscriminately, to cause suffering to the patient unnecessarily, is to commit the second fault in treatment.... A physician may become known to people living as far as one thousand miles by word of mouth, but he cannot be called a good physician unless he knows thoroughly about pulse diagnosis and human affairs; the way of treatment consists in the precious heritage of naturally established truth.... A physician who fails to administer treatment according to the established principles and forgoes the legitimate medical skills may treat his patients with effect by accident, but it is quite foolish for him to be content with his accidental success. Alas! Medicine is so subtle that no one seems able to know its complete secrets. The way of medicine is so wide that its depth is as immeasurable as the four seas. Unless you learn by heart, it is likely that you will remain in the dark about the bright theory of medicine.[71]

Sun Si-miao (581–682 A.D.), the greatest master of traditional Chinese medicine, stated the duties of a physician to his patients and to the public in the famous work *Bei Ji Qian Jin Yao Fang* (*Prescriptions Worth a Thousand Gold for Emergencies*):[72]

Medicine is an art which is difficult to master. If one does not receive a divine guidance from God, he will not be able to understand the mysterious points. A foolish fellow, after reading medical formularies for three years, will believe that all diseases can be cured. But, after practicing for another three years, he will realize that most formulae are not effective. A physician should, therefore, be a scholar, mastering all the medical literature and working carefully and tirelessly.

A great doctor, when treating a patient, should make himself quiet and determined. He should not have covetous desire. He should have mercy on the sick and pledge himself to relieve suffering among all classes. Aristocrat or commoner, poor or rich, aged or young, beautiful or ugly, enemy or friend, native or foreigner, and educated or uneducated, all are to be treated equally. He should look upon the misery of the patient as if it were his own and be anxious to relieve the distress, disregarding his own inconveniences, such as night-call, bad weather, hunger, tiredness, etc. Even foul cases, such as ulcer, abscess, diarrhoea, etc., should be treated without the slightest antipathy. One who follows this principle is a great doctor, otherwise, he is a great thief.

A physician should be respectable and not talkative. It is a great mistake to boast of himself and slander other physicians.

Lao-tzu, the father of Taoism, said, 'Open acts of kindness will be rewarded by man while secret acts of evil will be punished by God.' Retribution is very definite. A physician should not utilize his profession as a means for lusting. What he does to relieve distress will be duly rewarded by Providence.

He should not prescribe dear and rare drugs just because the patient is rich or of high rank, nor is it honest and just to do for boasting.[73]

## Greek Medicine: Aristotle

The Greek philosopher Aristotle (384–322 B.C.) studied under Plato, later tutored Alexander the Great, and finally founded the Peripatetic School in the Lyceum at Athens. His thought has stamped itself on the whole subsequent course of the biological and medical sciences, and indeed of all sciences. He laid the basis of the doctrine of organic evolution. He developed coherent theories of generation and heredity, and contributed greatly to embryology. Although Aristotle founded the science of comparative anatomy, he never used the human body itself as the material in his many animal dissections.

Like the earlier theory of the humors, Aristotle's theory held that there were four primary and opposite fundamental qualities, hot and cold, wet and dry. These met in binary combination to constitute the four essences, or elements, which entered in varying proportions into the constitution of all matter. The four elements were earth, air, fire and water. Water was wet and cold; fire was hot and dry; air was hot and wet; earth was cold and dry.

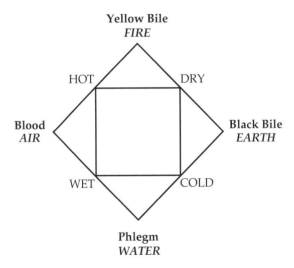

There is a similarity between Aristotle's theory and the Five Elements theory that has been acknowledged and practiced by Chinese philosophers and physicians for thousands of years. Five Elements theory was first recorded in the Chinese classic *Zuo Zhuan* (*Tso Chuan*, the famous commentary by Tso Chiu Ming on

*The Spring and Autumn Annals*) in 722 B.C., about four centuries prior to Aristotle's time.

## Roman Medicine

In Roman times, the Greek physician Galen (130–200 A.D.) made the most important contributions to medicine. His writings compiled the best of classical medicine, and this was the form in which medicine was transmitted through the medieval period to the Renaissance. Galen is considered the Father of Experimental Medicine because he developed the first theories of anatomy and physiology based on scientific experiments. However, because his knowledge of anatomy was based largely on animal experiments, he developed many false notions about the human body; many of his erroneous theories guided doctors for hundreds of years.

## The Middle Ages and Renaissance

The period of medicine as a science of observation closed with Galen. As the Roman Empire gradually disintegrated, European medical writers merely compiled the works of former authors. However, medical advances in Europe during the Middle Ages included the founding of many hospitals and the first university medical schools. Several important medical schools developed in Europe after the 11th century, and during the 11th and 12th centuries many of these schools became part of newly founded universities, such as the University of Bologna and the University of Paris.

The Muslim Empire of Southwest and Central Asia contributed greatly to medicine during the Middle Ages (about 200 A.D. to the 16th century A.D.). Rhazes, a Persian-born physician of the late 9th and early 10th century, wrote the first accurate descriptions of measles and smallpox. Avicenna, an Arab physician of the late 10th and early 11th century, produced a vast medical encyclopedia called *Canon of Medicine*. It summed up the medical knowledge of the time and accurately described meningitis, tetanus, and many other diseases. The work became popular in Europe, where it influenced medical education for more than 600 years. Islamic medicine had an impact on the Chinese as well. Among the achievements of Islamic medicine (Huiyi) introduced into China during the Yuan Dynasties were Huihuiyaowu (Islamic herbs), Huihuishiwu (Islamic foods), Huihuiyiyuan (Islamic hospitals) and Huihuiyaoqu (Islamic pharmacies).[74]

In the new scientific spirit that developed during the Renaissance (in Western Europe from about 1200 to 1600 A.D.), laws against dissection were relaxed, and the first truly scientific studies of the human body began. During the late 15th and early 16th century, Leonardo da Vinci performed many dissections to learn more about human anatomy. He recorded a series of more than 750 drawings. Andreas Vesalius (1514–1564), a physician and professor of medicine at the University of Padua in Italy, also performed many dissections and described several organs for the first time. Originally a Galenist, he became a leader in the revolt against Galen. His most important work, *On the Structure of the Human Body* (1543), was a scientific textbook on human anatomy which gradually replaced the texts of Galen and Avicenna.

### Modern Medicine

The Englishman William Harvey (1578–1657) performed many experiments in the early 17th century to learn how blood circulates. In 1676, the Dutch microscopist Anton van Leeuwenhoek (1632–1723) first observed what were later recognized as bacteria. Subsequent work by the German pathologist Rudolf Virchow (1821–1902) and the French microbiologist and chemist Louis Pasteur (1822–1895) ultimately led to the germ theory of disease.

The first practical anesthetic was introduced in 1842. Although physicians had tried to dull pain during surgery by administering alcoholic drinks, opium, and various other drugs for thousands of years, no drug had proved really effective in reducing the pain and shock of operations. Then two Americans, the physician Crawford Long (1815–1878) and the dentist William Morton (1819–1868), independently discovered that ether gas could safely be used to put patients to sleep during surgery. With this discovery, doctors could perform operations never before possible.

The concept of homeostasis is very important for contemporary Western medicine.[75] One of its earliest European roots can be found in the writings of an early 19th century German by the name of Kieser (1779–1862), who believed that any living thing was controlled by two forces, Yin and Yang. If the two forces balanced, then a normal vibration would take place and good health could be maintained. If one force became stronger than the other and blocked normal vibration, illness would result. Kieser is important because he may be one of the earliest modern Western medical scholars to apply the concepts of Yin and Yang.

Claude Bernard (1813–1878), the greatest 19th century French physiologist, discovered that the body maintains itself in a constant state with respect to temperature, acidity, hydration, salts, oxygen, and wastes. He defined the very important concept "milieu interieur" (internal environment) and indicated that to keep the internal environment constant is the primary condition for life's freedom and independence. In the words of Claude Bernard: "all the vital mechanisms, however varied they may be, have only one object [i.e., result], that of preserving constant the conditions of life in the internal environment."[76] Cannon (1871–1945) developed this concept, and in 1926 defined a new term, homeostasis, which means maintenance of static or constant conditions in the internal environment. Norbert Wiener (1894–1964), a great mathematician and the founder of cybernetics, developed this concept further, and discovered that the mechanism of control and regulation of homeostasis is negative feedback.[77]

In homeostasis, we can see a principle common to both Western and traditional Chinese medicine. The ancient Chinese medical classic *Nei Jing* emphasized that normal physiological activity can only be maintained when a relative balance is kept among the various internal organs, and between these organs and the external environment. Once this balance and coordination is lost, disease sets in. It stated that maintaining a relative equilibrium through the good, even development of Yin and the solidity of Yang would guarantee good health:

> The essentials of Yin and Yang are such that Yang energy should remain in solid state; a disharmony between Yin and Yang is comparable to spring without autumn or winter without summer; and to strike a balance between Yin and Yang is the way of the Sages.... When Yin is even and well while Yang is firm, the spirits will remain in proper order; divorce of Yin and Yang will cause the end of one's life.[78]

Franz Anton Mesmer (1734–1815), who studied medicine at Vienna, believed in "animal magnetism," an inner force that could be transferred from one organism to another. Healing could take place when a doctor either touched the patient softly or concentrated his consciousness on the patient. While Mesmer erred in mystifying the natural force, his idea was similar to the Chinese concept of **Chi** (Qi: vital energy, functional activities, breath, life force).

## Summary

The above is a brief historical account of Western medicine from the time of ancient Greece until the latter half of the 19th century when Western medicine was introduced into China. Before the 19th century there were many different theories and great advances in Western medicine, but there was never a consolidated medical system based on a unified theory, descending in a continuous line and practiced by all physicians. Many Western medical theories were derived from an anatomical view that was incomplete or faulty, or was based on subjective supposition, and therefore not of much value in diagnosis.

This is quite different from the development of traditional Chinese medicine. Although diverse schools of thought had also appeared in the course of development of Chinese medical science, all the basic theories could be traced to the *Nei Jing*, which originated from *I Ching* principles. Theories concerning the inner organs, channels (meridians), Chi and blood, body fluid and other physiological studies, and the pathological studies of heat and cold, excess and deficiency, proper Chi and harmful Chi, were set up at the time when the *Nei Jing* was written, and developed along the same line for more than two thousand years until the Qing Dynasty (1644–1911 A.D.). Although many of those theories require hypothesis and inference on the physician's part, diagnosis and clinical treatment are all based on an overall analysis of the illness and the patient's condition and are guided by a system of theories recognized by the various schools of thought in the medical field.[79]

# CHAPTER 10
# The Core of Traditional Chinese Medicine

## Yin Yang

Yi (first tone, means medicine) and Yi (fourth tone, means change) are based on the same principle.[80] *Nei Jing* stated that:

> The ancient people who knew the proper way to live followed the pattern of Yin Yang which is the regular pattern of heaven and earth, and remained in harmony with numerical symbols which are the great principles of human life.[81]

For the treatment of illnesses, one must understand the principles of the Yin Yang changes. Long long ago, Chinese acupuncturists studied the *I Ching* and discovered principles which have been integrated into acupuncture. For example, when a patient cannot move his arm, medicine based on Western science may treat only the shoulder joint, while Chinese medicine looks at the whole body. Based on the theory of Yin Yang balance, an acupuncture treatment might stimulate a point on the leg in order to affect the arm. For a headache, the needle might be put in the foot. If the patient's mind is relaxed, the treatment can help a great deal, and shortly after insertion of needles, pain disappears or movement is restored to the limb. Yin Yang theory also indicates acupuncture treatment for such conditions as mild strokes, where a person's center is lost and the whole body is affected, and in recent years acupuncture has been used for anesthesia, internal medicine and immunity. Students who understand and know how to practice Yin Yang theory will become good doctors of traditional Chinese medicine. Chinese culture and Western science are different from each other, like a circle and a square. One is not better than the other, just different. If you choose to study Chinese medicine, you need a strong foundation in the theoretical ground of Chinese culture. Only with a deep under-standing of both systems can a true integration between East and West be achieved.

General Aspects of Yin Yang

As we have seen, the Yin Yang idea is present in all the important Chinese texts, including the major classics of Confucianism and Taoism. Therefore, we could say that Yin Yang philosophy is the most important concept in common throughout Chinese culture.

> The Yin Yang doctrine is very simple but its influ-ence has been very extensive. No aspect of Chinese civilization—whether metaphysics, medicine, gov-ernment, or art—has escaped its imprint. In simple terms, the doctrine teaches that all things and events are products of two elements, forces, or principles: Yin, which is negative, passive, weak, and destruc-tive, and Yang, which is positive, active, strong, and constructive.[82]

Yin and Yang can refer to any complementary pair; for ex-ample, internal/external, intangible/tangible, spiritual/material, cold/hot, male/female, contracting/expanding, motion/rest, or inhale/exhale. It is important to realize that these pairs are not opposites, but rather the two extremes of the same process or quality: inhale/exhale are alternating extremes of breathing, cold and hot are poles of temperature. Yin and Yang exist in relation to each other and need each other to exist: we cannot have north without south; we feel heat in relation to something less hot. Yin and Yang each contains the essence of its complement. All things are composed of the two opposing elements; one wanes as the other waxes, yet they are ultimately and essentially complementary. If one loses its being, the other cannot exist either. That is why we say the single Yin will not live, and the lonely Yang will not grow. It takes Yin and Yang to create life, and only when the two are harmonized will there be a moral way. If one of the two antithetical elements is developed to the full, it may turn out to become the other element. For example, if one makes three left turns in succession, one ends up facing right. If one flies continuously toward the east, one ends up flying west. Therefore we say, if a thing is pushed to the extreme it is bound to produce counter effects; and when misfortune runs its course, fortune will come. If you desire a long and full life, you must neither overexert yourself nor do too little. The "golden mean" is the course you must follow.

As pictured in the Taichi diagram, Yin holds a small circle or seed of Yang, and Yang holds the seed of Yin. When Yin reaches its fullest extreme, it can change to Yang, and vice versa, so that there is a continual oscillation between the poles.

With terms such as passive or destructive, there may be cultural associations that lead to value judgements which are actually not present in Yin Yang theory in its pure form. Actually, Yin and Yang are value-free, relative positions, like the positive and negative poles of a magnet, rather than positive and negative in the sense of good and bad. Because Yin and Yang are symbols, we can use them to represent many things, from immediate situations to the most universal concepts. The table on the next page suggests some of the infinitely possible divisions of Yin and Yang into categories.[83] Remember that these categories are just conceptual guidelines, not literal divisions.

Yin and Yang can be defined as the two principles of female and male, in the sense that Yin and Yang are the elements that cause everything to grow and to develop. (Remember that Yin and Yang are like x and y, just symbols, so Yang does not stand

|                               | Yin              | Yang            |
| ----------------------------- | ---------------- | --------------- |
| Time                          | Night            | Day             |
| Temperature                   | Cold             | Hot             |
|                               | Coolness         | Warmth          |
| Gender                        | Female           | Male            |
| Weight                        | Heavy            | Light           |
| Season                        | Autumn, Winter   | Spring, Summer  |
| Brightness                    | Dark             | Light           |
| Motion                        | Downward         | Upward          |
|                               | Inward           | Outward         |
|                               | Relative Stasis  | Evident Motion  |
| Parts of the body             | Abdomen          | Back            |
|                               | Lower            | Upper           |
|                               | Zang (Tsang):    | Fu:             |
|                               | Viscera          | Bowels          |
| Activity, Function            | Blood            | Chi             |
|                               | Construction     | Defence         |
|                               | Calm             | Agitation       |
|                               | Weakness         | Strength        |
|                               | Passive          | Active          |
|                               | Contractive      | Expansive       |
|                               | Responsive       | Aggressive      |
|                               | Negative         | Positive        |
| Pulse                         | Slow             | Rapid           |
|                               | Deep             | Floating        |
|                               | Rough            | Slippery        |
|                               | Vacuous          | Replete         |
|                               | Small & Fine     | Large & Surging |
| Diagnosis                     | Yin disease      | Yang disease    |
| Cold/Heat                     | Cold             | Heat            |
| Exterior/Interior             | Interior         | Exterior        |
| Insufficiency/Excessiveness   | Shortage         | Excess          |
| Nature                        | Moisture         | Dryness         |
|                               | Rain             | Fire            |
| Wuxing (Five Elements)        | Metal            | Wood            |
|                               | Water            | Fire            |
| Flavors                       | Sour             | Sweet           |
|                               | Pungent          | Bitter          |
|                               | Salty            | Bland           |
| Numerology                    | Even             | Odd             |
| Computer binary code          | 0                | 1               |

just for man and Yin just for woman.) Yin and Yang tend to develop, respectively, in opposite directions; thus all living things
will eventually arrive at death. When descending Yin and as-
cending Yang separate, there arises a condition comparable to
the *I Ching* hexagrams Pi Gua (Hexagram 12, "Stagnation") or
the Wei Ji Gua (Hexagram 64, "Before Completion").[84] The character Pi means negative, denied, or regression, so Pi Gua is the
symbol of reversal. Wei Ji means unaccomplished, not successful,
so Wei Ji Gua is the symbol of what is not yet effected.

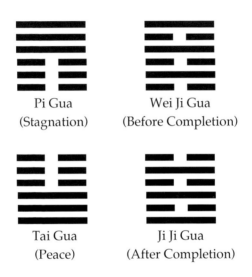

Pi Gua            Wei Ji Gua
(Stagnation)     (Before Completion)

Tai Gua           Ji Ji Gua
(Peace)          (After Completion)

The most important aspect of the Yin Yang principles involves
unification and harmony. This is the high wisdom that cultivates
balance between Yin and Yang, arriving at a state of unification or
neutralization. The situation where "Yin is even and well while
Yang is firm" is described in the *I Ching* hexagrams Tai Gua
(Hexagram 11, "Prospering, Peace"), the symbol of success, and
Ji Ji Gua (Hexagram 63, "After the End, or After Completion"),
the symbol of accomplishment, completion and consummation.[85]
The relationship between Yin and Yang is intergenerating as well
as mutually restricting; only through this kind of relationship can
harmony and unification be maintained.

We can apply the principles of Yin Yang in observing the phenomena of nature. For example, regarding the concept of time:

> Therefore it is maintained that there is Yin within Yin, and there is Yang within Yang. From dawn until noon is the period of Yang of Heaven; this is Yang within Yang. From noon until sunset is the period of Yang of heaven; this is Yin within Yang. From sunset until the crowing of the cock is the period Yin of heaven; this is Yin within Yin. From the crowing of the cock until dawn is the period of Yin of Heaven; this is Yang within Yin. The same applies to the human body.[86]

This cycle of Yin and Yang is expressed in a theory called the Principle of Midday/Midnight. You can apply the Yin Yang for-

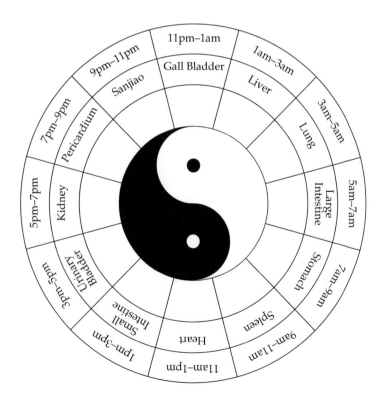

mula to any function or activity using this principle, for example sex. 11 a.m. to 1 p.m. is the peak of Yang within Yang, the time when the sun (Tai Yang) is at its height. Within the body, the heart is Yang within Yang (Yang/Yang). When energy goes to the heart, this is a time to avoid too much alcohol, sex, and so forth. At dawn, energy goes to the lungs and we need to get up and get fresh air; sex is not good at this time either. From observing the natural phenomenon of the rotation of the earth, we derive the principle that within Yin and Yang, there is also a Yin Yang change. The basis of the interacting and interchanging principles is that not only within the Yin is there a Yin and within the Yang a Yang; but even further, within the Yin there is a Yang and within the Yang a Yin. This allows for a complete interchange to occur. Therefore the study of Yin and Yang recorded in the *I Ching* and the *Nei Jing* is not a recognition of mere mechanics. The table below is an example of this principle in human physiology: women have male as well as female hormones, and men have female as well as male hormones.

| Sex Hormones (mg/ml) | Yin/Estrogens | Yang/Androgens |
|---|---|---|
| | (estradiol) | (testosterone) |
| Yin/Women | $0.07^a$–$0.17^b$ | 0.5 |
| Yang/Men | 0.024 | 6.5 |

[a]Follicular phase of the menstrual cycle (sexual cycle)
[b]Luteal phase of the menstrual cycle (sexual cycle)[87]

The utilization of Yin Yang theory is unlimited. Let us briefly review some further applications:

Anatomy and Physiology

> When Yin and Yang are applied to man, the external regions belong to Yang, and the internal regions belong to Yin. When Yin and Yang are applied to the human body, the back belongs to Yang, and

|                                      | Yin                    | Yang                     |
| ------------------------------------ | ---------------------- | ------------------------ |
| body                                 | interior               | outer                    |
|                                      | back                   | front                    |
|                                      | top                    | bottom                   |
| body system                          | maintenance system     | control system           |
| movement system                      | flexion                | extension                |
|                                      | relaxation             | contraction              |
| respiratory system                   | inspiration            | expiration               |
| cardiovascular system                | diastole               | systole                  |
| digestive system                     | ingestion              | defecation               |
|                                      | absorption             | digestion                |
| metabolism system                    | anabolism              | catabolism               |
| reproductive system genetic code     | XX                     | XY                       |
| gonads                               | ovaries                | testes                   |
| sex hormones                         | estrogens              | androgens                |
|                                      | estradiol              | testosterone             |
| sexual organ                         | clitoris               | penis                    |
|                                      | labium major           | scrotum                  |
| nervous system brain                 | inhibition             | excitation               |
| autonomic                            | parasympathetic        | sympathetic              |
| endocrine system pancreas            | insulin                | glucagon                 |
| hypothalamus                         | inhibitory hormones    | releasing hormones       |
| parathyroid                          | parathyroid hormones   | calcitonin               |
| control mechanism                    | negative feedback      | positive feedback        |

the abdomen belongs to Yin. When Yin and Yang are applied to the viscera and bowels, the viscera belong to Yin and the bowels belong to Yang. The liver, the heart, the spleen, the lungs and the kidneys are the live viscera, and they all belong to Yin; the gall bladder, the stomach, the large intestine, the small intestine, the bladder, and the San Jiao (Triple Warmer) are the six bowels and they belong to Yang. Why do we need to know Yin within Yin and Yang within Yang? For example, the back belongs to Yang, and the heart is the Yang within the Yang. The back belongs to Yang and the lungs are the Yin within the Yang. The abdomen belongs to Yin, and the kidneys are the Yin within the Yin. The abdomen belongs to Yin, and the liver is the Yang within the Yin. The abdomen belongs to Yin, and the spleen is the extreme Yin within the Yin. These are the descriptions of the correspondence between Yin and Yang of the human body and the Yin Yang of Heaven.[88]

This utilizes the principles of Yin and Yang in the classification of the organs in the human body. This is how we begin to look at the exterior and interior of the human body, the characteristics of the internal organs, and the relationship between the viscera and the bowels, using the principles of Yin and Yang. These principles coincide with the Yin Yang principles of the universe and support the saying that Heaven and Man are one. In terms of modern human physiology, there are many further associations with Yin and Yang, as illustrated on the facing page.[89]

Pathology

In a healthy body, the relationship between Yin and Yang is harmonious, balanced, and unified. The internal supporting strength of Yin depends on the external defending functions of Yang, and development of the defending functions of Yang, in turn, relies on the support of the internal strength of Yin. If the Yang Chi is overly strengthened and cannot close, the Yin Chi will be weakened and the relationship between Yin and Yang will be severed. When Yin and Yang separate, then **Jing** (essence) will be exhausted; all sorts of regressive actions will start, similar to the ones described in the *I Ching*, and illness will develop, creating a chance for external factors to invade and harm the body.

If Yin and Yang are unbalanced in the body, then signs of illness will show up on the side of the weaker of the two. Also,

> Severe cold will produce heat and severe heat will produce cold.[90]

When Yang becomes stronger, symptoms such as heat arise; if Yin becomes stronger, symptoms of cold arise. However, severe cold will bring about the false appearances of heat, and severe heat will bring about the false appearances of cold. Severe Yin turns into Yang and severe Yang turns into Yin. This pathological change fits in well with the principles of the interchanging of Yin and Yang. In the diagnosis of diseases, this is of extremely great value.

When the external defense function becomes weakened in the Yang, the outer surfaces of the body will "fear" cold. The Yin Chi then becomes deficient and damaged and false heat will arise within the body. When there is an excess of Yang, the whole body will feel feverish. Where there is an excess of Yin, a false cold will arise from within the body. This gives us a new view of a pathological problem from the reverse side.

> Where the vicious energy attacks, the true Chi will be deficient.[91]

When all the symptoms that cause illness gather together and attack the living substance, then the body must be in a state where harmony is lacking and the Yin and Yang are unbalanced. First the true Chi becomes weakened, then disease breaks out. The factors that can cause a disease are caused by something from either within the body or outside of it. This is what we mean by saying that the vicious energy may be derived from the Yin or from the Yang. Wind, rain, cold, or summer heat are external causes; diet imbalance, living habits, and inability to control emotions are internal causes.

## Diagnosis

For a practitioner of traditional Chinese medicine, there are various ways of diagnosing disease:

1. Diagnosis from outer appearance: the ancient people believed that whenever illness occurred, and when there were changes within the human body, it would reflect on the coinciding places on the surface of the body, thus causing a change in form and expression.
2. Diagnosis by listening: from the sounds of the patient's voice, its high or low pitch, strength or weakness; the way the patient breathes, whether the breath is fine, slow or intense, the doctor can determine where the illness lies.
3. Diagnosis by asking questions: employing various means to find the answers to the questions enables the doctor to determine the cause of the disease and the symptoms.
4. Diagnosis by contact: this includes taking the pulse and by touching the skin, abdomen, arms or legs of the patient. There are two kinds of pulse-taking, one at the wrist and one at different parts of the body.

Regardless of the method used, the most important point is to remember that one should first differentiate between Yin and Yang. Next observe the outer appearance and ascertain the internal feelings, then the insubstantial and substantial, cold and heat, etc. Only after all of this can one make an appropriate diagnosis.

A good diagnostician will observe the patient's complexion, take his pulse, and take the first step in determining if it is a Yin disease or a Yang disease. He will examine the patient's complexion to

| Examination | Yin Signs | Yang Signs |
|---|---|---|
| Looking | Quiet, withdrawn, slow, frail manner; patient is tired and weak, likes to lie down curled up; no spirit; excretions and secretions are watery and thin; tongue material is pale, puffy, and moist; tongue moss is thin and white. | Agitated, restless, active manner; rapid, forceful movement; red face; patient likes to stretch when lying down; tongue material is red or scarlet, dry; tongue moss is yellow and thick. |
| Listening & Smelling | Voice is low and without strength; few words; respiration is shallow and low and patient is weak; shortness of breath; acrid odor. | Voice is coarse, rough, and strong; talkative; respiration is full and deep; putrid odor. |
| Asking | Feels cold; reduced appetite; no taste in mouth; desires warmth and touch; copious and clear urine; pressure relieves discomfort; scanty pale menses. | Patient feels hot; dislikes heat or touch; constipation; scanty, dark urine; dry mouth; thirst. |
| Touching | Frail, minute, thin, empty, or otherwise weak pulse. | Full, rapid, slippery, wiry, floating, or strong pulse. |

see if it is clear or muddy in order to locate the internal organ affected; he will observe the patient's
panting and breathing, hear his voice, in order to

identify the patient's suffering; he will take the pulse focusing on the pulses of the four seasons, namely, falling pulse for winter, light and floating pulse for autumn, smooth pulse for spring, forceful pulse for summer, in order to determine which internal organ is affected; he will take the pulse at the wrist to see if it is a superficial pulse, or a deep pulse, or a sliding pulse, or a retarded pulse, in order to know the nature of disease and treat it accordingly; and when the diagnosis is not erroneous, treatment will not fail to produce effects.[92]

As the following recent text shows, the patterns of Yin and Yang signs are still the basis of diagnosis in contemporary practice of traditional Chinese medicine.

Yin and Yang disharmonies are the most general, all-inclusive patterns in Chinese medicine. Indeed, all the patient's symptoms may ultimately be reduced to whether the pattern of the individual's illness is Yin or Yang. Yin patterns are combinations of signs associated with Interior, Deficiency and Cold, while Yang patterns are woven from signs appropriate to Exterior, Excess, and Heat.[93]

Some of these relationships are enumerated in the table on the facing page.

Treatment

Treatment is based on an overall analysis of symptoms and signs, including the cause, nature and location of the illness and the patient's physical condition, as determined according to the basic theories of traditional Chinese medicine. The goal of therapeutic treatment is to control the imbalances and to strengthen the weaknesses in the human body in order to achieve harmony between Yin and Yang within the living organism and allow it to remain healthy and strong.

> Generally speaking, cold patterns are treated by warming, heat patterns by clearance, vacuity patterns by supplementation, and repletion patterns mostly by precipitation.[95]

> A cold disease should be heated up, a hot disease should be made cold, a warm disease should be cooled down, a cool disease should be warmed up, a dispersing disease should be constricted, an inhibiting disease should be dispersed, a dry disease should be lubricated, an acute disease should be slowed down, a hard disease should be softened, a crisp disease should be hardened, a weakening disease should be toned up, a strong disease should be sedated.[96]

## Diet and Diet Therapy

As early as the *Nei Jing*, Chinese medical doctors included nutrition and diet therapy as an important aspect of health and medical care.

> Medicinal herbs can attack diseases, the five grains can nourish the body, the five fruits can assist the five grains in nourishing the body, the five domestic animals' meat can benefit the body, the five vegetables can fill up the needs of the body; thus energies and flavors can combine forces to tone up the 'jing' (essence of life) and 'qi'.[97]

In Western diet, foods are considered for their protein, carbohydrates, fats, calories, vitamins, minerals, and other nutrient content, but in traditional Chinese diet, foods are considered for their five flavors, five energies, movements, and common and organic actions. Yin Yang theory is the basis of nutrition and diet therapy in traditional Chinese medicine, which starts from the premise that we naturally like to eat foods that correct our particular imbalance. If we feel cold, we want to eat something that will warm us; if we're hot, we want something to cool us. Similarly, we naturally like to eat foods that strengthen our particular weakness; for example, someone who feels his or her kidneys weakening will want to eat something that will strengthen that function.

In traditional Chinese medicine, the body types, diseases, moods, and four seasons may be classified into Yin and Yang.[98] For example, one's body type may be hot (Yang), or cold (Yin); one's disease may be interior (Yin), or exterior (Yang). The nature and effect of herbs and foods may also be classified according to Yin and Yang. For example, cold, cool, rich, and moist agents are Yin, whereas warm, hot, dry, and fierce agents are Yang.

> Agents pungent and sweet in savor are Yang, while those that are salty, bitter, sour, or astringent in savor are Yin. Agents whose qi and savor are bland and mild are Yang, and those whose qi and savor are strong are Yin.[99]

Chinese medical science is extremely complex, but Yin Yang theory is the heart of it; if you understand Yin and Yang, your teeth will be strong enough to crack the nut of Chinese medicine.

### Wuxing (Five Elements)

The Theory of the Five Elements was first mentioned in *Shu Jing* (*The Book of History*).

The Nature of Wuxing:
Water tends to seep down
Fire tends to flare up
Wood tends to branch out
Metal cuts through the skin
Earth creates harvesting crops[100]

> First generated from Tu (Earth), then mixed with
> Jin (Metal), Mu (Wood), Shui (Water) or Huo (Fire),
> the substance would turn into a myriad things with
> life.[101]

If we want to comprehend theories of Chinese medicine, we must discuss not only Yin Yang theory but also the application of **Wuxing** (the Five Elements, Five Interactions, or Five Phases, shown below). The Theory of the Five Elements points out that water, fire, wood, metal and earth are the basic energies constituting the material world. Here we shall mention the interpromoting and the interrestricting (nurturing and destroying) relations of the Five Elements. Their interpromoting and interrestricting interactions are diagrammed on the facing page).

Wuxing theory has been a simple and widely-used tool from ancient times in China, and it has a mysterious side to it. From description of physiological functions, to understanding of patho-

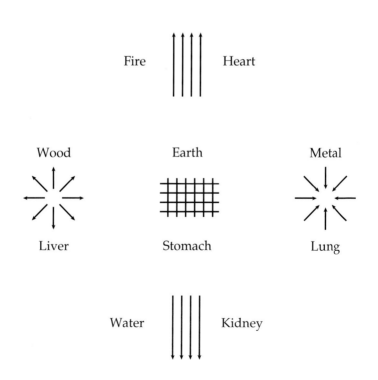

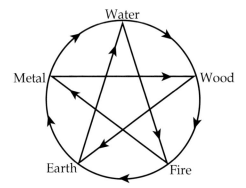

logical changes, to diagnosis and treatment of diseases, the implementation of Wuxing has been common and popular. For example, in terms of the physiological functions of the five internal organs, Wuxing theory is used to depict the relationship between them, either strengthening, weakening or counter-acting. In explaining the pathological changes of the organs, the theories of creating, controlling, acting or counteracting effects of Wuxing are emphasized. In explaining how climate affects pathological changes of the internal organs, we again have to turn to the theories of Wuxing.

In Chinese philosophy, Wuxing theory is both function and foundation. The Wuxing are simply five symbols representing existing phenomena; we could use less metaphorical and evocative symbols, like A, B, C, D, and E. One can use Five Elements theory any time, since everything contains the five energies. Is this a desk? No—it's wood...but it isn't wood, it's a tree...but it's also earth, and water. Everything contains the interrelated and interdependent Five Elements. We are aware that Wuxing theory originated from and cannot be separated from Yin Yang theory, so we can conclude that Wuxing is Yin Yang, and Yin Yang is Tao.

In contemporary terms, the Chinese philosophical thought expressed as "Heaven and Man are one" means "Apply the laws of nature and its ways of change to the study of humankind." People are a part of nature. There are things we cannot explain because human physiology and psychology, like nature itself, are complex, profound, and still obscure. Five Element theory can be a useful tool in understanding nature and ourselves.

> Heaven has four seasons and Five Elements, which on the one hand are in control of birth, growth, harvest and storage, and on the other in control of producing cold, heat, dryness, humidity and wind. The five viscera in man are capable of producing five energies, which in turn are responsible for the five emotions of joy, anger, sadness, grief and fear.[102]

In nature, we have the four seasons, spring, summer, autumn and winter. Spring belongs to wood, summer to fire, autumn to metal, long summer (usually translated as Indian Summer) to earth, and winter to water. Spring and summer mark the strengthening of the reproductive and growth functions, while autumn and winter preserve the function of formation. This then becomes the regular pattern of nature. The internal organs would function likewise. Heart, liver, spleen, lungs and kidney matched up with Wuxing would become fire, wood, earth, metal and water respectively; from these would derive the five emotions. With the above theory we are able not only to discern the application of Yin and Yang in the process of symbiosis, interacting and counteracting, but also to observe the relationship between people and nature. In diagnosis and treatment, this knowledge is very important.

From the interpromoting and interrestricting relations of Wuxing, we know that comparable relations exist among the five internal organs. The effects of the Wuxing on the four seasons and the five internal organs can give us an idea of this relationship between them. Chapter 10 of the *Nei Jing*, "Growth of the Five Viscera," outlines the connections between the heart, liver, spleen, lungs, kidney and various other parts of the body, such as blood vessels, skin, tendons, muscles and bones, and clearly explains the inter-promoting and inter-restricting relation between each one. We can judge the nutrition in the body by observing the complexion, body hair, nails, lips and head hair. Generally speaking, Yin and Yang and the Five Elements are physiologically balanced. The interpromoting and interrestricting relationships act only as needed for retaining balance. If one element becomes stronger than the rest, a person's health is harmed.

The *Nei Jing*[103] describes Five Element theory in terms of the effect of emotions, climate and diet on the organs of the body and their functions. Liver functioning is disrupted when one becomes very angry, although feeling sorrow can lessen the anger. In terms of climate, damp wind can harm the tendons and cause liver trouble, but dryness can create balance. A diet with too much sour food can harm the tendons and the liver, while acrid and hot food can overcome this condition. Heart disease is related to emotional imbalance manifested as excessive joy or exhilaration, which can be lessened by fear; extreme heat, which can be overcome by coolness; or too much bitter food, which can be overcome by saltiness. Traditional Chinese doctors consider the pancreas as belonging to the spleen, functioning to regulate the blood and help digestion. The major emotional cause of spleen disease is seen as disruption of the digestive system caused by obsessive thinking, which can be stopped by the emotion of anger. High humidity and dampness harms the spleen and the flesh, which also relates to the spleen, but ventilation decreases the dampness in the air. Sweet foods harm the flesh and spleen, but sour foods or herbs can overcome the effects of excess sweet. Extreme grief harms the lungs, but happiness can counteract the grief. Hot weather and acrid foods can harm skin and hair, which are associated with the lungs, but cold and bitter can prevail over heat. Fear is harmful to the kidneys, but contemplation can calm the fear. Intense cold is sufficient to harm the blood and kidneys, but dry heat can overcome the cold. Salt can do harm to the blood and the kidneys, but sweet can overcome the salt.

From the time of the *Nei Jing*, traditional Chinese medicine has approached diagnosis from a holistic point of view, consid-

| Category | Five Elements | | | | |
|----------|------|------|-------|-------|-------|
|          | Wood | Fire | Earth | Metal | Water |
| **Nature** | | | | | |
| Season | Spring | Summer | Indian Summer | Autumn | Winter |
| Climate | Wind | Heat | Damp | Dryness | Cold |
| Development | Germination | Growth | Transformation | Reaping | Storing |
| Colors | Cyan | Red | Yellow | White | Black |
| Tastes | Sour | Bitter | Sweet | Pungent | Salty |
| Direction | East | South | Center | West | North |
| **Human Body** | | | | | |
| Yin Organ | Liver | Heart | Spleen | Lung | Kidney |
| Yang Organ | Gall Bladder | Small Intestine | Stomach | Large Intestine | Urinary Bladder |
| Sense Organ | Eye | Tongue | Mouth | Nose | Ear |
| Tissue | Tendons | Vessels | Muscle | Skin | Bone |
| Emotions | Anger | Joy | Pensiveness | Sorrow | Fear |
| Expression | Yell Grasp | Laugh Grieve | Sing Nag | Cry Cough | Moan Tense |
| Affecting | Spleen (earth) | Lung (metal) | Kidney (water) | Liver (wood) | Heart (fire) |
| **Mind** | Benevolence | Faith | Politeness | Justice | Intelligence |
|          | Soul | Mind | Idea | Spiritedness | Will |
|          | Humanity | Authenticity | Reason | Wisdom | Faith |

ering emotions, climate and diet as well as the symbiotic and interacting theories of the Five Elements. This system has had long-lasting effects on the development of Chinese medical science. The illustration on the facing page lists some categories of the Five Elements.


## Jingluo (Meridians)

**Jingluo** (channels, or meridians) is one of the most important and unique concepts in traditional Chinese medicine. In this theory, there exists within the human body a system of channels through which the Chi and blood circulate, and by which the internal organs are connected with superficial organs and tissues and the body made an organic whole. The points on the body surface are the particular spots where the vital energy of the internal organs reaches. When one is ill, the physician can regulate the patient's flow of vital energy by puncturing certain points on his body surface and thus cure the illness of the associated internal organs.[104] The three illustrations that follow indicate the fourteen primary channels.[105]

The channels are based on the Yin Yang and Five-Elements theories of the body. For example, from the names of twelve of the primary meridians, one can see that the channels combine aspects of Yin and Yang and the Five Elements.

Blood is carried through the meridians by Chi, nourishing and protecting the body and helping maintain its functions. The channels are like lines of communication among the various parts of the body. When an acupuncture needle is used on a healthy person, there is a sensation that the channel is alive with energy. When a person is ill or injured, symptoms may appear that relate to the external course of the channel or to an internal organ associated with that channel. A skilled practitioner of traditional Chinese medicine knows how to select acupuncture points on the basis of Yin Yang correspondence among the primary channels and organs, points of intersection among the meridians, special

| 1.  | Arm Greater Yin     | Lung channel             | (Hand Taiyin)   |
|-----|---------------------|--------------------------|-----------------|
| 2.  | Arm Yang Brightness | Large Intestine channel  | (Hand Yangming) |
| 3.  | Leg Yang Brightness | Stomach channel          | (Foot Yangming) |
| 4.  | Leg Greater Yin     | Spleen channel           | (Foot Taiyin)   |
| 5.  | Arm Lesser Yin      | Heart channel            | (Hand Shaoyin)  |
| 6.  | Arm Greater Yang    | Small Intestine channel  | (Hand Taiyang)  |
| 7.  | Leg Greater Yang    | Urinary Bladder channel  | (Foot Taiyin)   |
| 8.  | Leg Lesser Yin      | Kidney channel           | (Foot Shaoyin)  |
| 9.  | Arm Absolute Yin    | Pericardium channel      | (Hand Jueyin)   |
| 10. | Arm Lesser Yang     | Triple Burner channel    | (Hand Shaoyang) |
| 11. | Leg Lesser Yang     | Gall Bladder channel     | (Foot Shaoyang) |
| 12. | Leg Absolute Yin    | Liver channel            | (Foot Jueyin)   |

characteristics of individual points, cutaneous regions and the broad domains of the connecting channels.

There is one great Taichi circle containing many Yin Yang circles: the human body with its meridians contains many Taichi circles, and each channel contains Yin and Yang and the Five Elements. By practicing awareness of Yin and Yang, regular Taichi exercise, and opening yourself, you can truly understand the meridians and points and become a good doctor of traditional Chinese medicine.

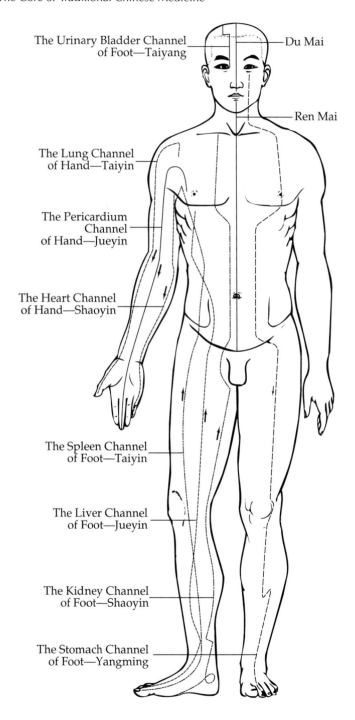

The Urinary Bladder Channel of Foot—Taiyang

Du Mai

Ren Mai

The Lung Channel of Hand—Taiyin

The Pericardium Channel of Hand—Jueyin

The Heart Channel of Hand—Shaoyin

The Spleen Channel of Foot—Taiyin

The Liver Channel of Foot—Jueyin

The Kidney Channel of Foot—Shaoyin

The Stomach Channel of Foot—Yangming

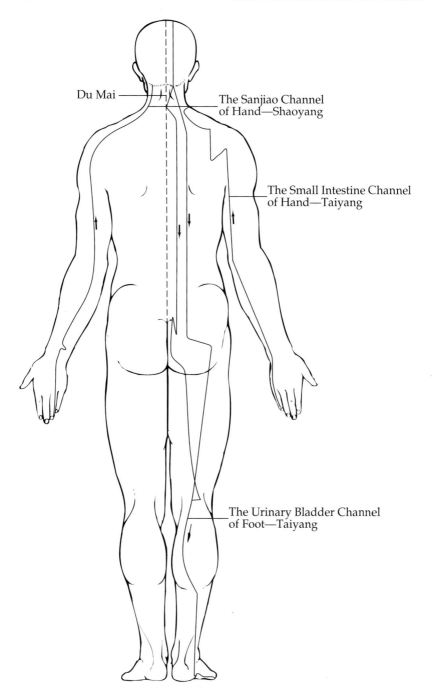

Du Mai

The Sanjiao Channel
of Hand—Shaoyang

The Small Intestine Channel
of Hand—Taiyang

The Urinary Bladder Channel
of Foot—Taiyang

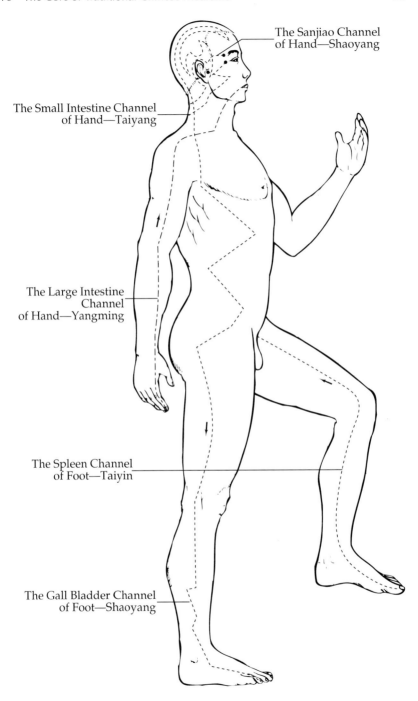

The Sanjiao Channel
of Hand—Shaoyang

The Small Intestine Channel
of Hand—Taiyang

The Large Intestine
Channel
of Hand—Yangming

The Spleen Channel
of Foot—Taiyin

The Gall Bladder Channel
of Foot—Shaoyang

# CHAPTER 11
# The Taichi Philosophy and Its Applications

## Taichi Philosophy

The Taichi symbol gives us a model of the relationship between Yin and Yang, and between the parts (Yin and Yang) and the whole (the Taichi circle). The Taichi circle is absolute, while each part, Yin or Yang by itself, is relative. The balance of the relative parts creates the absolute circle: Three into One. Since Yin and Yang are relative, their interactions can be very complicated. Relativity needs to be understood because although the absolute does not exist in the same tangible, perceptible, or measurable way as its relative manifestations, the absolute contains and is made apparent by the balanced relatives.

If we call Yin and Yang time and space, the circle is energy. If we call Yin and Yang 1 and 2, the circle is 3. Taichi and Yin Yang, the absolute and the relative, are integral to each other, Three into One. We can use this Taichi philosophy to guide the practice of Chinese medicine, acupuncture, Chi Kung, Taichi Chuan, Taichi nutrition and diet therapy, and Taichi meditation, as well as to conceptualize the broad subjects of culture, religion, and philosophy. Taichi shows us that the One generates Yin and Yang, which combine in infinite manifestations. Some of these are expressed in such paradigms as the Five Elements and the Eight Trigrams. The Taichi philosophy, or Taichimonism, permeates all aspects

| Yin | Yang | Taichi |
|---|---|---|
| One | Two | Three |
| Negative part | Positive part | Circle |
| Negative extreme | Positive extreme | Zhong (The Golden Mean) |
| Material Culture | Social Culture | Spiritual Culture |
| First-Level Culture | Second-Level Culture | Third-Level Culture |
| Things | Persons | Thoughts |
| Money | Power | Heart (Spirit) |
| Disease | Health | Homeostasis |
| Female | Male | Love |
| Person A | Person B | Friendship |
| Universe | Human Being | Tao |
| Breath | Action | Emptiness |

of life, culture, and universe. The table above and subsequent discussions show just a few of the ways this metaphor can be applied.

## Applications of Taichi Philosophy

Meditation

In meditating, one balances one's own Yin and Yang, whether it is termed $X$ and $Y$, 0 and 1, self and other, sun and moon, or good and bad. Everything in the world is changing, but the meditator is aware of the continual change from Yin to Yang, Yang to Yin, as constant as the alternation of day and night.

The meditator is conscious of these great forces which control and form the universe by their constant flux, and in their combined operation form the Tao, the Way, the great principle of the universe.

Imagine a man who is so ill that medical treatment can't cure him. He's a rich man, but he cannot be satisfied by material things. Other people can't help him find peace. Nothing on the material or societal levels can heal him, so he empties his mind

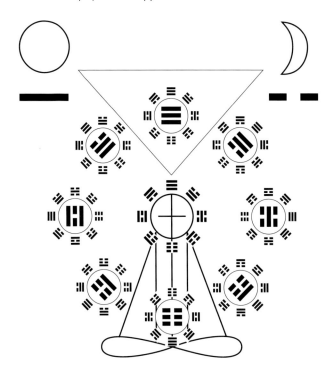

and goes beyond his troubles. This is meditation. Looking for something eternal, the meditator's mind is open. Only change is eternal, not fleeting. Faith in this principal is the key, the essential ingredient for understanding. This faith brings the strength of spirituality, the strength of the third level of culture. Because the open mind is relaxed, it may seem crazy, stupid, or childlike, but it is actually strong and creative.

Meditation is a way of spiritual development as well as a means to better health. The state of consciousness associated with meditation does not occur spontaneously. It is induced by ancient techniques developed over centuries by practitioners of various spiritual traditions. Meditation is a set of techniques producing a rested, relaxed body and an aware, relaxed mind, thereby permitting the development of a "higher consciousness." Most forms of meditation involve being still and focusing, emptying the mind of distractions, or concentrating on one thought or object.

A relaxed open mind is extremely beneficial for physical and mental health. Several recent studies have shown that meditation produces striking physiological changes along with those feelings generally reported and considered important to meditators. Meditators show both highly specific EEG patterns and prominent changes in body functioning. Although alpha waves are normally produced only when an individual's eyes are closed, in the case of the meditators alpha waves appear in their EEGs even with their eyes open. Oxygen consumption drops sharply shortly after meditation begins. A blood substance normally associated with anxiety and hypertension shows a marked decrease during meditation. Wallace and Benson, noted researchers of meditation, suggest that in fast-paced industrial societies like the United States, meditation might well be used to help people relax and maintain their psychological equilibrium.[106]

Presently there are many different methods of meditation in the United States. The meditation of traditional Chinese culture is what we define as Taichi meditation, which is not a religious practice, but an activity based on Yin Yang and Wuxing theory. Within the scope of Taichi meditation are included such practices as Taichi sitting, Taichi chanting, Taichi walking, Taichi exercise (Taichi Chuan, Chi Kung, etc.), Taichi breathing, Taichi diet, and Taichi healing. The goal is the improvement of one's physical and mental health through Yin Yang balance. Of particular importance to students of this form of meditation is concentration on Taichi breathing. The more you practice, the greater the possibilities for opening and self-cultivation.

Remember that in Taichi, Yin and Yang are relative, and easier to see, discuss, and regulate than the abstract concept of the circle. If you understand 1 and 2, you can control 3. This is the basis of the Taichi meditation mind. Because the absolute is an abstraction that cannot be comprehended in concrete terms, we need an open mind to understand it. To practice meditation is to learn the subconscious activity of self-control in a natural way.

A meditation master cannot open other meditators' minds for them, but can point out a direction and hope they will understand. Your body is your temple. Meditation can open you to what can be called God, emptiness, breath, or whatever you sincerely believe. Rather than a religion, this is a belief system based on the notion that Sincerity is One, and One is Sincerity. When empty, you can open to what is, and discover the nature of existence. The trouble is that it is not easy for people to open. Yin and Yang are everywhere, but each individual needs to find a Way to balance them. This can be achieved through empty mind. Emptying the mind is difficult. An empty mind is a clear mind, not hollow or blank. When you experience something with an empty or open mind, you can remember it easily, like a song you heard when you were first in love. Open your mind, respect yourself, and approach everything with sincerity.

Exercise and Posture

The practice of Taichi Chuan can permit one to open more readily. Our bodies have their own form of eternity: breath. Without breath, there is no life, no time or space. Teaching breathing is a good way to teach Yin and Yang. Since everyone can breathe already, many people may not think they need a teacher. To learn Taichi Chuan is to experience the Yin and Yang of inhale and exhale. Physical action contains the principle of Yin and Yang as well. Therefore, breath and physical action together constitute Yin Yang balance. The Yin and Yang of mind cannot be talked about directly, but people can be taught how to use movement and breathing together to empty the mind. Action and breathing together, mind empty, Three into One, is Taichi. This is something to practice with sincerity every day.

**Chi Kung, Kung Fu and Taichi exercise are presently very popular in China and other countries, including America. The principle of integration of Three into One (action, breathing, and concentra-**

**tion/emptiness) is essential to Chi Kung. Please
note that practicing Chi Kung without understanding this basic principle may cause imbalance between body and mind, between Yin and Yang.**

In contemporary terms, Yin Yang theory represents both the
psychological and the physiological states—they cannot be separated. Inhale represents Yang, and exhale represents Yin. Breathing that balances Yin and Yang carries balance to the body's systems. To the practitioner of Taichi breathing, inhaling can include
concentrating on the intergenerating cycle of the Five Elements:
wood (liver) promotes fire (heart), strengthening earth (spleen),
which generates metal (lungs), promoting water (kidney), nourishing wood, and so forth. Exhaling, the conscious mind cou-
ples with the intercontrolling and counteracting functions of the
different substances, resulting in metal (lung) overcoming wood
(liver), which then quiets earth (spleen), controlling water (kidney), calming fire (heart). Both interactions can balance Yin and
Yang to promote health of body, mind, and spirit.

Physical sensations are relative to the individual and hard to
communicate. If you taste something and find it sweet, the best
way to describe that sensation to other people is to have them
taste and experience it for themselves. Similarly, through deep
Taichi exercise, one can have a direct experience of Yin and Yang,
the Five Elements, Chi, and other intangible aspects which might
otherwise seem merely theoretical. Because of this, students who
learn and practice Taichi Chuan can be better doctors. Taichi, like
meditation, has to be experienced individually; however, once it
has been perceived directly, the experience can be shared with
others.

Taichi Chuan is like the Taichi symbol on the opening page
of Chapter 1. The physical and energetic center of the body, just
below the navel, is called the **Dan Tien** (Dan Tian, Field of Elixir)
which can be compared to the One (Taichi, Grand Ultimate). All
of the Taichi Chuan movements originate from this center, just
as the One generates Yin and Yang (Liang Yi, the Two Modes).

Taichi breathing is inhaling and exhaling from the center, and the Taichi form balances the parts of the body that are above and below the center, right and left, front and back, and so forth. Taichi movements continuously shift the body's weight and energy from empty to full. The arms and legs become the Four Forms (Si Xiang). The Eight Trigrams are found in the joints: shoulder, elbow and wrist, hip, knee and ankle, and two important places in the upper and lower spine. By moving from the center with the spine erect, coordinating breathing with movement, and concentrating the mind on the breath, the Taichi practitioner creates Yin Yang harmony. Taichi balances Yin and Yang. Mind, breath and action are Three into One.

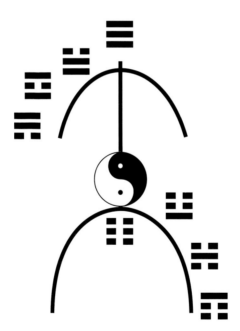

The continuous and varied evolution of the trigrams develop the innumerable forms of Taichi Chuan. Sincerity is the essential principle underlying the practice of Taichi Chuan. We can easily see external Yin Yang balance by looking at a person's posture.

There is also a less obvious internal Yin Yang balance, similar to the concept of homeostasis, which can be achieved by practicing Taichi Chuan with sincerity and openness.

In the classroom or office, as in meditating, straight posture and correct gesture create a sense of rightness and sincerity. Sitting in a state of balance keeps the center open. If you are balanced, standing or sitting, you have Chi; if you are not balanced, there is no Chi. People say that after sitting a long time they need to slouch or to shift their weight around to help their circulation. If you have to do this, you do not have balance of Yin and Yang, and you need to learn to regulate your breath. If you have good breath, you can sit with one center. If you sit off-centered, first the kidney meridian lines are affected, and then the other Yin meridians of the legs, the spleen and the liver. Chi goes up the leg, affects your lower spine, then you get a sore neck. Develop good sitting habits, and practice exercise such as Taichi Chuan to stretch the meridians. When you develop Chi you can sit for a long time.

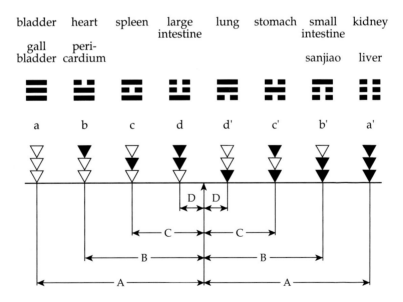

Studying and Practicing Medicine

To become a doctor of Chinese medicine, the student needs to master a 5,000-year-old culture. A doctor who is too attached to either Western science or Eastern philosophy will not approach patients with a clear mind. To achieve a clear mind, the doctor needs to be in balance with the patient by constantly trying to balance his or her own Yin and Yang. For example, in order to check a patient's pulse, you need to be centered and to concentrate. Make the patient's hand comfortable, then make your own hand relaxed, sit correctly, and breathe from your center. The patient's Yin and Yang are invisible. You won't discover this principle by simply reading about it in a book.

If you visit my clinic, you will see me using Yin Yang theory to help patients. For example, many people are very frightened of acupuncture needles and therefore are difficult to treat. I instruct such patients that when I say yes or no, they should say the opposite. Yes/No; Yes, yes/No, no; No, no, yes, no/Yes, yes, no, yes. I only insert the needle when the patient's mind has yes/no balance and is therefore relaxed and empty.

A patient came to me who had inoperable cancer. Someone who has been told by a doctor that he has cancer starts to worry, and this may develop into a heart problem. This patient had watched his mother die a painful death from cancer. His brother, a heart specialist himself, had a heart condition and had recently undergone triple bypass surgery. Science can be of great benefit, and I sometimes use information obtained through Western science and medical testing to aid in my own diagnosis of certain patients. But in this case I didn't have access to this patient's medical records. I used the traditional Chinese method of diagnosis: with an empty mind I checked his pulses and understood the patient internally. This is a way of applying the Yin/Yang/Taichi formula of inside/outside/both together (Three into One). I understood from his pulses that his condition was serious. I didn't want to lie to him—I told him he might die. His other doctors had already told him he had only months to live and had already signed the forms for him to go to the hospital. His insurance would cover the costly procedures they prescribed to briefly prolong his life. The recommended treatment was chemotherapy and radiation; this is strong poison. Many of the Chinese herbs used to cure cancer are natural poisons, but these medicines have not been approved by the U.S. government. This is a difficult kind of patient to take on, since it would be risky to claim I could cure him.

In this case I studied the entire family, assessing the medical history of each member and the nature of their relationships as a family. I arranged a meeting with the patient and the family members who played the most important roles in his life, his two daughters and his son. I asked them: does your home have a tiger? I explained that the illness of their father was the tiger, and that I would go to meet the tiger but I didn't know who would win. After this meeting and an initial treatment of acupuncture and herbs, I left him and let him decide for himself whether he wished to continue treatment with me. Although I might be eaten by the tiger, I knew that a doctor can't decide for the patient. This patient had strong trust in me. He and his family believed that his cancer was terminal but they put their faith in me to save him.

I used especially strong and often poisonous herbal medicines. The family understood this treatment might not be effective in this case. I rarely talked with the patient about the treatments. Instead, he and I discussed the tiger. After a series of treatments, the patient began to feel better. Finally I asked him an important question. If he could provide the answer, I could guarantee he would recover. The question was about an imaginary animal, a combination of lion and dragon, a meat eater, fiercer than a tiger. There is a bell hanging around its neck. The question was: how can you remove the bell without killing the animal or yourself? If he could solve this question, I could cure him with herbs.

The patient was able to find a new calmness and quiet in his life. Every day he thought about the question; every day he rang the bell, even in his dreams he would still ring the bell. When

I told some of my students about this question, they asked if the animal was asleep, to which I answered it pretended to be. The students had quick solutions to this deep question, such as the need to lose your fear, or to make friends with the animal. However, the animal doesn't care if you're afraid of it or not, it will kill you anyway. People without cancer can play with this question, but the cancer patient lives this question every day. I cooked herbs for him every day. But he caught cold and needed oxygen, which necessitated his going to the hospital. The nurses asked him why he seemed so calm even though he was dying of cancer. He answered, "Every day I ring a bell." Moments before his death he told me, "I'm sorry, I'm dying and I still cannot answer the question." I'm not God; I could not save him. He died calmly, ringing the bell.

Every day this bell rings in my office. I still treat this man's family. Whenever I think about that man and the bell, I am with him and I smile. This kind of story can be useful in treating a critically ill patient. Help him remain open and peaceful, and from inside he can heal. The daughter recently visited me. She said she always thinks about the question but still can't answer it. Perhaps you don't have cancer, and you don't feel the need to know this story. But we each need to teach ourselves, and to open our minds.

**Balance and Harmony**

To go a step further, the Taichi philosophy may be applied comprehensively, in all human relationships, whether on an individual, a national, or a world level.

Relationships

A single individual is just one point. When another person comes along, another point is added, forming a line. Two extremes, Yin

and Yang, are not easy to keep balanced. There are always con-
tradictions, conflict, and struggle between them. Only by adding
a third point will the line become a balanced triangle. The third
point here does not represent another person. It is the intangible:
God, Tao, Sincerity, Love, Respect, Good, Spirituality, the Third
Level of Culture or, in short, the Taichi Circle. The invisible third
point is the basis of balance between the two persons.

In some cases, the third point forming the triangle may be a
third person. More and more points form endless relationships
of triangles, expanding out in all directions, as below. It is hard
to find the center, but using the Taichi metaphor can help in
bringing concepts back to what is simplest and most basic, similar
to the way 6/2 can be reduced to 3/1 in mathematics. Always
remember Yin Yang and Taichi. Always use the spiritual qualities
of the Taichi Circle to regulate and balance Yin and Yang, to
work through your hangups, to open your mind, to guide your
exercise, to strengthen your mental and physical well-being, to
seek and enjoy happiness.

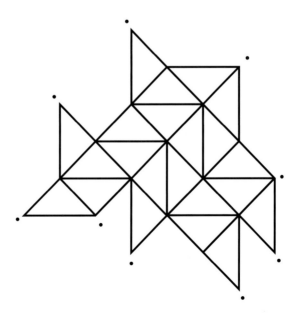

In mathematics, a point has no dimension. The two points shown here represent two separate individuals, without any relationship to each other. This corresponds to the first, or material, level of culture.

The two points are connected by a line. They communicate with each other, corresponding to the second level of culture, but a line in mathematics still only represents one dimension.

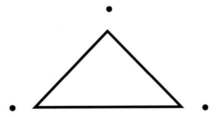

Three points define a plane. Adding the third point makes a triangle, which is stable but still abstract.

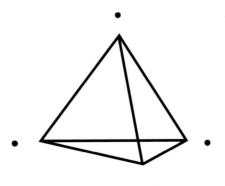

Adding a fourth point, we can suggest a three-dimensional figure. The third level of culture is not visible—we need faith. The top point of the pyramid represents spirit.

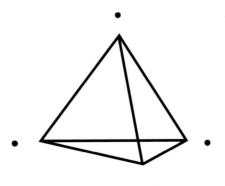

Like the Taichi symbol, these diagrams are an indirect way of describing something of an intangible spiritual nature—we can only point toward the ultimate, the absolute.


## World Culture

We can use the Taichi philosophy to look at the world at large. In terms of the Wuxing, East is wood, West is metal, North is water, South is fire, and the center is earth. Metal penetrates wood, wood permeates earth, earth contains water, water extinguishes fire, and fire melts metal. In terms of Yin Yang balance, there is too much of the metal element (penetrating or centripetal force) in the West, evidenced by weaponry and technological science. If carried to excess, the piercing metal element leads to destruction. If the Asian (East—wood element) and American (West—metal element) powers come into balance, then balance could follow between Russia (North—water) and the Third World (South—fire), resulting in the possibility of global harmony.

The world and its inhabitants are all interrelated and form a coherent entity. Whether individual or nation, all are One. As in the

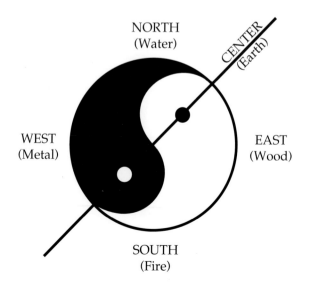

Taichi circle, all are equal: One divides into Two (Yin and Yang). The world is divided into East and West or South and North, developed and developing nations, and so forth, while people are divided into rich and poor, educated and uneducated, male and female, and so forth. One and Two unite into Three. Three transcends One and Two, beyond politics, religion, and science; it is a very simple and broad philosophical outlook. This, the essence of the third level culture, the spiritual in human beings, is contained in the Taichi model.

Even as the spirits of great musicians such as Mozart, Beethoven, and Chopin live on through the people who play and listen to their music, the spirits of great sages such as Lao-tzu, Confucius, Jesus, and Sakyamuni stay alive in our hearts through their greatest teachings. Their breath is carried on by us, and our breath will be carried on in turn by our children. We respect our ancestors as their spirits are still with us, and we hope our children will remember us in spirit as well.

Not all that exists is material. Not all that lives is physical. Not all that has meaning is science. Not all that has spirit is religion. Through sharing and communicating with each other, we can strive toward Yin Yang balance and spiritual harmony, transcending time and space.

# Notes

1. D.C. King and M.R. Koller, *Foundations of Sociology*, (San Francisco: Rinehart Press, 1975), pp. 46–47.

2. Li-fu Chen et al., *An Introduction to Chinese Culture*, (Taipei, Taiwan: The Council of the Chinese Cultural Renaissance, 1977), p. 5.

3. Mu Qian, *Essays on Chinese Culture*, Book I, (Taipei, Taiwan: Sanming Books Co., 1973), p. 2.

4. By Henry C. Fenn, 1958; cited in Clarence Burton Day, *The Philosophers of China: Classical and Contemporary*, (Secaucus, NJ: The Citadel Press, 1978), pp. 409–410.

5. A latest measure reported in *People's Daily*, October 23, 1989, Overseas Edition.

6. Chen, p. 7.

7. Hunan Provincial Museum and Institute of Archeology, Academia Sinea, *The Han Tomb No. 1 at Mawangtui, Changsha*, (Peking: Wenwu Press, 1973), p. 40.

8. Wing–tsit Chan, *A Source Book in Chinese Philosophy*, (Princeton, NJ: Princeton University Press, 1963), p. 262.

9. A. Colin Ronan and Joseph Needham, *The Shorter Science and Civilisation in China: I*, (Cambridge: Cambridge University Press, 1978), p. 180.

10. Chan, p. 262.

11. Translation of *I Ching*, The Great Appendix: Section I, Chapter 11, in Chan, p. 262.

12. Translation of *I Ching*, The Great Appendix: Section I, Chapter 5, in Chan, p. 266.

13. Translation of *I Ching*, The Great Appendix: Section II, Chapter 6, in Chan, p. 268.

14. Cited by Chao Chen: "Yi and Medicine," *The Studies of the Application of The Book of Changes*, Vol. II, ed. Li-fu Chen et al, (Taipei, Taiwan: Chung Hwa Books Co., Ltd., 1982), p. 439.

15. Book II, Chapter 5: Great Treatise on Yin Yang Classifications of Natural Phenomena. Henry C. Lu, trans., *A Complete Translation of the Yellow Emperor's Classic of Internal Medicine and the Difficult Classic*, (Vancouver, Canada: The Academy of Oriental Heritage, 1987), p. 30.; and Ilith Veith, trans., *The Yellow Emperor's Classic of Internal Medicine*, (Berkeley, CA: University of California Press, 1972), p. 115.

16. Clarence Burton Day, *The Philosophers of China: Classical and Contemporary*, (Secaucus, NJ: The Citadel Press, 1978), p. 30.

17. Day, pp. 31–32.

18. Day, pp. 30–32 and 49; and Li-fu Chen, pp. 14–17.

19. Some historians, such as Charles O. Hucker in his *China's Imperial Past: An Introduction to Chinese History and Culture* (Stanford, CA: Stanford University Press, 1975), divide Chinese history into the following periods: the Formative Age, Prehistory–206 B.C., the Early Empire, 206 B.C.–960 A.D., and the Later Empire, 960–1850.

20. Frederic H. Chaffee et al., *Area Handbook of Communist China*, (Washington D.C.: U.S. Government Printing Office, 1967), p. 241.

21. Chin-Hua Chou, "New Explanation of Midday and Midnight Law in Accupuncture," (*China Medical College Annual Bulletin*, vol. 7, 1976), pp. 58 and 107.

22. *Li Ji* (*The Book of Rites*), Chapter 9: "Li Yun (Evolution of Li)."

23. In 1894, James Legge translated this quotation as: "To enjoy food and delight in colors is nature." And in his note, he added that: "We might suppose that 'se' here denoted 'the appetite of sex.' But another view is preferred."—James Legge, trans., *The Works of Mencius* Book VI, *Kao Tsze* Part I, Chapter 4, (New York: Dover Pub., Inc., 1970), p. 397.

Here 'se' should mean sex, not color.

24. Chen, p. 35–36.

25. Chen, p. 37–38.

26. Chan, p. 107.

27. Chan, pp. 136–137.

28. Stephen Mitchell, *Tao Te Ching*, (New York: Harper and Row, 1988), p. 25.

29. Mitchell, p. 42.

30. Wen-Shan Huang, *Fundamentals of Tai Chi Ch'uan*, (Hong Kong: South Sky Books Co., 1984), p. 74.

31. Chen, pp. 40–41.

32. Chaffee et al., p. 242.

33. Yen-nien Wang, *Tai Ji Quan: Yang Family Hidden Tradition, An Explanation through Photos*, (Taipei, Taiwan: The Grand Hotel Tai Chi Chuan Association, 1988), p. H-7; and Huang Wen-shan, *Fundamentals of Tai Chi Ch'uan*, (Hong Kong: South Sky Books Co., 1984) pp. 52–65.

34. Day, p. 95.

35. Day, p. 97

36. Chan, p. 336.

37. This translation is based on: D. T. Suzuki, "English translation of the Shingyo," in *Manual of Zen Buddhism*, (New York: Grove Press, 1960), pp. 26–30; and Edward Conze, "The Heart Sutra: Sanskrit Text, Translation and Commentary," in *Buddhist Wisdom Books*, (London: George Allen and Unwin, 1958), pp. 76–107.

38. There are two versions of the Heart Sutra: the one printed above is the shorter sutra in general use in China and Japan. The larger text, which includes opening and concluding passages, may be found in *Manual of Zen Buddhism* by D. T. Suzuki, pp. 27–28.

39. Conze, pp. 76–107.

40. This illustration comes from a woodprint by Giichi Minoshima, in *Living a Simple Life Through Zen*, (The Institute for Zen Studies, 1984), p. 1.

41. See Chan and Day for fuller descriptions of the Chinese Buddhist Schools.

42. D. T. Suzuki, cited in Chan, p. 425.

43. John C.H. Wu, *The Golden Age of Zen*, (Taiwan: United Publishing Co., 1967), p. 44.

44. Chan, p. 425.

45. Wu, p. 31.

46. Wu, p. 60.

47. Wu, p. 62.

48. This is a condensation of Wu, Chapter IV, "Hui-Neng's Fundamental Insights," p. 75–80.

49. *The Sutra of Hui-neng*, cited and translated in Wu, p. 85. Hui-neng is the only sacred Chinese Buddhist writing to be honored with the rank of Jing (classic or sutra).

50. This translation is based on Mitchell, p. 1; Chan, p. 139; and Zi-chang Tang, *Wisdom of Dao*, (San Rafael, CA: T.C. Press, 1969), p. 206.

51. Wu, p. 86.

52. *The Sutra of Hui-neng*, cited and translated in Wu, p. 79.

53. Wu, p. 89.

54. Ji-yu Ren, ed., *Zhong Jiao Cidian* (*Dictionary of Religion*), (Shanghai: Shanghai Cishu Press, 1985), pp. 936, 1016, 840.

55. Paul H. Clyde and Burton F. Beers, *The Far East: A History of The Western Impact and the Eastern Response (1830–1970)*, (Englewood Cliffs, NJ: Prentice Hall, 5th ed., 1971), pp. 56–57.

56. Clyde and Beers, p. 161.

57. J. Mason Gentzler, ed., *Changing China: Readings in the History of*

*China from the Opium War to the Present,* (New York: Praeger Publishers, 1977), pp. 43–44.

58. Clyde and Beers, p. 86.

59. Gentzler, p. 62.

60. "Taizu you Dao, Dao yu Shangdi tongzai, Dao jiushi Shangdi," *The New Testament (Revised Standard Version and Kuoyu [Mandarin] Union Version),* (Taiwan: The Bible Societies in Republic of China, 1974), p. 257; *The New Chinese Bible (New Testament),* (Hong Kong: The New Chinese Bible Commission), 1976, p. 129.

61. Stephen T. Chang, *The Great Tao,* (San Francisco: Tao Publishing, 1985), p. 15. See also Day, p. 315.

62. Yi Wu, *The Sincerity Philosophy of the Doctrine of the Mean,* pp. 16–18.

63. Z. D. Sung, *The Text of Yi King,* (Taipei, Taiwan: Jin-gang Press, 1986), p. 7, The Text: Section I:1. The Khien Hexagram.

64. Sung, pp. 7–8, The Text: Section I:1. The Khien Hexagram.

65. Li-fu Chen, *Si Shu Dao Guan (The Tao of the Four Books),* (Taipei, Taiwan: World Books, Co., 1966), pp. 242–262.

66. These page numbers were taken from: James Legge, trans., *The Four Books,* (Taipei, Taiwan: Culture Book Co., 1983).

67. These page numbers were taken from *The New Testament (Revised Standard Version and Kuoyu [Mandarin] Union Version),* (Taiwan: The Bible Societies in Republic of China, 1974).

68. Hong-Yen Hsu, *Chen (Chan-Yuan)'s History of Chinese Medical Science,* (Taipei, Taiwan: Modern Drug Publishers Co., 1977), p. 112.

69. See P.T. Marshall, *The Development of Modern Biology,* (Oxford, UK: Pergamon, 1969), pp. 58–93.

70. Norman Burke Taylor, ed., *Stedman's Medical Dictionary,* 19th revised ed., (Baltimore: The Williams and Wilkins Co., 1957), p. 652.

71. Henry C. Lu, *A Complete Translation of the Yellow Emperor's Classic,* Book X, Chapter 78: On Commiting Four Faults, pp. 633–635.

72. Sun Si-miao (652 A.D.), *Prescriptions Worth a Thousand Gold for Emergencies*, Reprint, (Beijing: People's Medical Publishing House, 1982), pp. 1–2.

73. Tao Lee, "Medical Ethics in Ancient China," *Bulletin of the History of Medicine*, **8** (3), (March 1943), p. 268–269.

74. Manqing Zheng and Pinshi Lin, *A History of Traditional Chinese Medicine*, (Taipei, Taiwan: Taiwan Commercial Press, 1982), p. 278.

75. Fang Fu Ruan, "Medicine in the Twentieth Century," *Journal of the Dialectics of Nature*, 7 (1), (1985), pp. 43–50.

76. A.J. Carlson and V. Johnson, *The Machinery of the Body*, 3rd ed., (Chicago: The University of Chicago Press, 1948), p. 78.

77. Fang Fu Ruan, "On the Historical Development of the Concept of Homeostasis," in *Progress in Physiological Sciences*, 11 (3), (1980), pp. 284–286; and "The Development of the Concept of Homeostasis," in *New Treatise on Medicine*, (Harbin: Heilongjiang Scientific and Technological Publishing House, 1984), pp. 52–63.

78. *Nei Jing*, Book I, Chapter 3: On the Correspondence of Life Energy with the Energy of Heaven. This translation is based on Lu, *A Complete Translation of the Yellow Emperor's Classic*, pp. 20–21; and Zhu-fan Xie and Xiaokai Huang, eds., *Dictionary of Traditional Chinese Medicine*, (Hong Kong: The Commercial Press, Ltd., 1984), pp. 2–3.

79. Tedao Jia, *A Short History of Traditional Chinese Medicine*, (Taiyuan, China: Shanxi People's Publishing House, 1979), p. 291.

80. Xue-xi Zhou, *Ten Lectures on the Study of Yi Jing*, (Chengdu, China: Sichuan Scientific and Technological Press, 1986), pp. 5–10.

81. *Nei Jing*, Book I, Chapter 1: On the Heavenly Truth of Ancient Times. Lu, p. 2.

82. Chan, p. 244.

83. See Manfred Porkert, *The Theoretical Foundations of Chinese Medicine*, (M.I.T. East Asian Science Series, vol. 3, 1982), pp. 22–31; and East Asian Medical Studies Society, *Fundamentals of Chinese Medicine*, (Brookline, MA: Paradigm Publications, 1985), pp. 19–20.

84. R. L. Wing, *The I Ching Workbook*, (Wellingborough, UK: The Aquarian Press, 1984), pp. 12 and 64.

85. Wing, pp. 11 and 63.

86. *Nei Jing*, Book I, Chapter 4: On the Ultimate Truth in the Emperor's Golden Bookcase. Lu, p. 24.

87. Fang Fu Ruan, *Discovery of the Sex Hormones*, (Beijing: Science Press, 1979), p. 113.

88. *Nei Jing*, Book I, Chapter 4. Lu, pp. 24–25.

89. Fang Fu Ruan, "Body Regulation and Yin-Yang Theory." Unpublished manuscript of lecture given on March 18, 1989, at ACCHS and Taoist Center, Oakland, California.

90. *Nei Jing*, Book I, Chapter 5. Lu, p. 40 and pp. 23–33.

91. *Nei Jing*, Book IX, Chapter 33. Lu, p. 380.

92. *Nei Jing*, Book II, Chapter 5. Lu, pp. 44–45.

93. Ted J. Kaptchuck, *The Web That Has No Weaver: Understanding Chinese Medicine*, (New York: Congdon and Weed, 1983), p. 184.

94. Kaptchuk, pp. 184–185.

95. East Asian Medical Studies Society, p. 449.

96. *Nei Jing*, Book IX, Chapter 74: Great Treatise on the Importance of Ultimate True Energies. Lu, pp. 590–591.

97. *Nei Jing*, Book VII, Chapter 22: On Energies of Viscera Responding to the Four Seasons. Translated by the author; see also Lu, p. 151.

98. Henry C. Lu, *Chinese System of Food Cures: Prevention and Remedies*, (New York: Sterling Publishing Co., Inc., 1986), p. 35.

99. East Asian Medical Studies Society, p. 9.

100. *Shu Jing* (*The Book of History*). Cited by Yu Mei-yin: "Yi and the Dao of Medicine," in *The Studies of the Application of The Book of Changes*, vol. I, Li-fu Chen et al., (Taipei, Taiwan: Chung Hwa Books Co., Ltd., 1981), p. 479.

101. *Guo Yu* (*Conversations of the States*). Cited by Yu Mei-yin: "Yi and the Dao of Medicine," in *The Studies of the Application of The Book of Changes*, vol. I, Li-fu Chen et al., p. 479.

102. *Nei Jing*, Book II, Chapter 5. Lu, pp. 33–34.

103. *Nei Jing*, Book II, Chapter 5: Great Treatise on Yin Yang Classifications of Natural Phenomena. Lu, pp. 36–40.

104. Zhu-fan Xie and Xiao-kai Huang, eds., *Dictionary of Traditional Chinese Medicine*, (Hong Kong: The Commercial Press, Ltd., 1984), p. 261.

105. The Cooperative Group of Shandong Medical College and Shandong College of Traditional Chinese Medicine, *Anatomical Atlas of Chinese Acupuncture Points*, (Jinan, China: Shandong Science and Technology Press, 1982), pp. 3–5.

106. A. Lazerson et al., *Psychology Today: An Introduction*, 3rd ed., (New York: CRM/Random House, 1975), pp. 296–297.

# References

Bible Societies in Republic of China. *The New Testament (Revised Standard Version and Kuoyo [Mandarin] Union Version)*. Taiwan: The Bible Societies, 1974.

Blofeld, John, trans. and ed. *I Ching (The Book of Change): A New Translation of the Ancient Chinese Text with Detailed Instructions for its Practical Use in Divination*. New York: E.P. Dutton and Co., Inc., 1968.

Capra, Fritjof. *The Tao of Physics*. 2nd Revised and updated ed. New York: Bantam, 1988.

Chaffee, Frederic H., et al. *Area Handbook for Communist China*. Washington, D.C.: U.S. Government Printing Office, 1967.

Chan, Wing-tsit, trans. and comp. *A Source Book in Chinese Philosophy*. Princeton, NJ: Princeton University Press, 1963.

——. "Taoism," in *Encyclopedia Britannica*. Volume 21, 1968.

Chang, Kwang-chih. *The Archaeology of Ancient China*. New Haven: Yale University Press, 1977.

Chang, Stephen T. *The Great Tao*. San Francisco: Tao Publishing, 1985.

Chao, C. *Belief in God in Ancient China*. Taipei, Taiwan: Chinese For Christ, Inc., 1976.

Chen, Chao. *Essence of Acupuncture Therapy as Based on Yi King and Computers*. Taipei, Taiwan: Fangong Press, 1976.

Chen, Li-fu. *Si Shu Dao Guan (The Tao of the Four Books)*. Taipei, Taiwan: World Books, Co., 1966.

————, et al. *An Introduction to Chinese Culture.* Taipei, Taiwan: The Council of the Chinese Cultural Renaissance, 1977.

————, ed. *Yixue Yinyong zhi Yanjiu (The Studies of the Application of The Book of Changes).* Vol. I. Taipei, Taiwan: Chung Hwa Books Co., Ltd., 1981.

————, ed. *Yixue Yinyong zhi Yanjiu (The Studies of the Application of The Book of Changes).* Vol. II. Taipei, Taiwan: Chung Hwa Books Co., Ltd., 1982.

————. *Dui Zhongguo Yiyao zhi Yuanwang (The Wishes for Chinese Medicine and Pharmacology).* Taizhong, Taiwan: Zhongguo Yiyao Xueyuan, 1987.

Ch'en, Kenneth K.S. *Buddhism in China: A Historical Survey.* Princeton, NJ: Princeton University Press, 1972.

Cheng, Man-jan. *Lao-Tzu: "My Words Are Very Easy To Understand."* Richmond, California: North Atlantic Books, 1981.

Cheng, Shao'en. *Zhongyi Yunqixue (The Studies on the Five Circuit Phases and the Six Atmospheric Influences in Traditional Chinese Medicine).* Beijing: Beijing Scientific and Technological Publishing House, 1986.

Chiang, Kung-cheng. *Yi Jing de Kexue Tixi (The Scientific System of I Ching).* Taipei, Taiwan: College of Chinese College, 1966.

Chou, Chih-hua. "New Explanation of the Midday and Midnight Law in Acupuncture." *China Medical College Annual Bulletin.* Vol. 7, 1976.

Chou, Chih-hua. *Zhenjiu yu Kexue (Acupuncture and Science).* 2d ed. Taipei, Taiwan: Qi-ye Books Co., 1987.

Clyde, Paul H. and Burton F. Beers. *The Far East: A History of the Western Impact and the Eastern Response (1830-1970).* 5th ed. Englewood Cliffs, NJ: Prentice-Hall, 1971.

Colegrave, Sukie. *Uniting Heaven and Earth.* Los Angeles: Jeremy P. Tarcher, Inc., 1979.

Conze, Edward. *Buddhist Wisdom Books.* London: George Allen and Unwin, 1958.

Creel, Herrlee G. *Chinese Thought from Confucius to Mao Tse-tung.* Chicago: The University of Chicago Press, 1953.

Day, Clarence Burton. *The Philosophers of China: Classical and Contemporary*. Secaucus, NJ: The Citadel Press, 1978.

East Asian Medical Studies Society, Wiseman, Nigel and Andrew Ellis, trans. *Fundamentals of Chinese Medicine*. Brookline, MA: Paradigm Publications, 1985.

Fu, Tong-sian. *Zhongkuo Huijiao Shi (A History of Islam in China)*. 2d ed. Taipei: Taiwan Commercial Press, 1972.

Fung, Yu-lan, Derk Bodde, trans. *A History of Chinese Philosophy*. 7th Printing. Princeton, NJ: Princeton University Press, 1973.

Gentzler, J. Mason, ed. *Changing China: Readings in the History of China from the Opium War to the Present*. New York: Praeger Publishers, 1977.

Giles, Herbert A. *Religions of Ancient China*. Folcroft Library Editions. London: Archibald Constable and Co., 1976.

Holbrook, Bruce. *The Stone Monkey: An Alternative, Chinese-Scientific, Reality*. New York: William Morrow and Co., 1981.

Hookham, Hilda. *A Short History of China*. New York: New American Library, Inc., 1972.

Hoover, Thomas. *Zen Culture*. New York: Vintage Books, 1978.

Hsu, Hong-Yen. *Chen (Chan-Yuan's) History of Chinese Medical Science*. William G. Peacher trans. Taipei, Taiwan: Modern Drug Publishers Co., 1977.

Huang Wen-Shan. *Fundamentals of Taichi Ch'uan*. 5th ed. Hong Kong: South Sky Books Co., 1984.

Institute for Zen Studies. *Living a Simple Life Through Zen*. Calendar. Kyoto, Japan: Hanazono College, 1984.

Jia, Tedao. *Zhongguo Yixue Shiluo (A Short History of Traditional Chinese Medicine)*. Taiyuan, China: Shanxi People's Publishing House, 1979.

Kaptchuk, Ted J. *The Web That Has No Weaver: Understanding Chinese Medicine*. New York: Congdon and Weed, 1983.

King, D.C. and Koller, M.R. *Foundations of Sociology*. San Francisco: Rinehart Press, 1975.

Lazerson, A. et al. *Psychology Today: An Introduction.* 3rd ed. New York: CRM/Random House, 1975.

Lee, T. "Medical Ethics in Ancient China." *Bulletin of the History of Medicine.* Vol. **8** (3), March 1943.

Legge, James, trans. *I Ching (Book of Change).* New York: University Books, Inc., 1964.

———. *The Four Books.* Taipei, Taiwan: Culture Book Co., 1983.

———. *The Works of Mencius.* New York: Dover Pub., Inc., 1970.

Long, Pojian. *Huangdi Nei Jing Gailun (An Introduction to the Yellow Emperor's Classic of Internal Medicine).* Shanghai: Shanghai Scientific and Technological Publishing House, 1980.

Lu, Gang-yong et al., eds. *Daozhang Qigong Shu Shizhong (Ten Books of Taoist's Collection and Chi-Kong).* Beijing, China: Traditional Chinese Medical Classics Press, 1987.

Lu, Henry C., trans. *A Complete Translation of the Yellow Emperor's Classic of Internal Medicine and the Difficult Classic.* Vancouver, Canada: The Academy of Oriental Heritage, 1978.

———. *Chinese System of Food Cures: Prevention and Remedies.* New York: Sterling Publishing Co., Inc., 1986.

Markert, Christopher. *I Ching: The No. 1 Success Formula (Let This Time-tested Method Help You Make The Right Decisions—Today).* Wellingborough, UK: The Aquarian Press, 1986.

Marshall, P.T. *The Development of Modern Biology.* Oxford, UK: Pergamon, 1969.

Matsumoto, Kiiko and Stephen Birch. *Five Elements and Ten Stems: NAN CHING Theory, Diagnostics and Practice.* Higganum, CT: Paradigm Publications, (no date).

Michael, Franz. *China Through the Ages: History of a Culture.* Boulder, CO: Westview Press, 1986.

Mitchell, Stephen. *Tao Te Ching.* New York: Harper and Row, 1988.

Needham, Joseph. "Sexual Techniques." In *Science and Civilisation in China.* Volume 2. Cambridge, UK: Cambridge University Press, 1954.

———. "Sexuality and the Role of Theories of Generation." In *Science and Civilization in China*. Volume 5. Cambridge UK: Cambridge University Press, 1983.

Paden, William E. *Religious Worlds: The Comparative Study of Religion*. Boston: Beacon Press, 1988.

Porkert, Manfred. *The Theoretical Foundations of Chinese Medicine*. M.I.T. East Asian Science Series, Vol. 3. Nathan Sivin, ed. Cambridge, MA: The M.I.T. Press, 1982.

———, with Dr. Christian Ullmann. *Chinese Medicine: Its History, Philosophy and Practice, and Why It May One Day Dominate the Medicine of the West*. Mark Howson, trans. Revised ed. New York: William Morrow and Co., 1988.

Qian, Mu. *Zhongguo Wenhua Congtan (Essays on Chinese Culture)*, Book I. Revised ed. Taipei, Taiwan: Sanming Books Co., 1973.

———. *Kongzi yu Lunyu (Confucius and the Analects)*. Taipei, Taiwan: Lianjing Publishing Co., (1st ed., 1974), 1975.

———. *Linghung yu Xin (Soul and Mind)*. Taipei, Taiwan: Lianjing Publishing Co., (1st ed., 1976), 1977.

———. *Cong Zhongguo Lishi Lai Kan Zhongguo Minzushen ji Zhongguo Wenhua (Understanding Chinese Nationality and Chinese Culture Based on Chinese History)*. Taipei, Taiwan: Lianjin Publishing Co., (1st ed., 1979), 7th reprinting, 1985.

Ren, Ji-yu, ed. *Zhong Jiao Cidian (Dictionary of Religion)*. Revised edition. Shanghai: Shanghai Cishu Press, 1985.

Ronan, A. Colin and Joseph Needham. *The Shorter Science and Civilisation in China: I*. Cambridge: Cambridge University Press, 1978.

Ruan (Juan), Fang Fu. *Sheng Ji Su de Fa Xian (Discovery of the Sex Hormones)*. Expanded 2d ed. Beijing: Science Press, 1983.

———. *Yi Xue Xin Lun (New Treatise on Medicine)*. Harbin: Heilongjiang Scientific and Technological Publishing House, 1984.

———. *Xingxue yu Yixue (Sexology and Medicine)*. Hong Kong: Genius Publishing Co., 1989.

Schuon, Frithjof. *In the Tracks of Buddhism.* Marco Pallis, trans. 1st ed., 1968. London: Unwin Paperbacks, 1989.

Shandong Medical College and Shandong College of Traditional Chinese Medicine, The Cooperative Group. *Anatomical Atlas of Chinese Acupuncture Points.* Jinan, China: Shandong Science and Technology Press, 1982.

Shanghai College of Traditional Medicine. *Acupucture: A Comprehensive Text.* J. O'Connor, trans. and D. Bensky, ed. 5th printing. Seattle, WA: Eastland, 1987.

Shi, Xianyuan et al., eds. *Zhongguo Wenhua Zhi Mi (The Enigmas of Chinese Culture).* 3 vols. Shanghai: Xielin Press, 1985, 1987, 1988.

Sun Si-miao. *Bei Ji Qian Jin Yao Fang (Prescriptions Worth a Thousand Gold for Emergencies).* Reprint. Beijing: People's Medical Publishing House, 1982.

Sung, Z.D. *The Text of Yi King (And Its Appendixes): Chinese Original with English Translation.* Revised ed. Taipei, Taiwan: Jin-gang Press, 1986.

Suzuki, Daisetz Teitaro. *Essays in Zen Buddhism.* 2d ser. Boston: The Beacon Press, 1952.

———. *Essays in Zen Buddhism.* 1st ser. New York: Grove, 1961.

———. *Manual of Zen Buddhism.* New York: Grove Press, 1960.

———. *Studies in Zen.* Chinese Translation Edition, Men Xiangshen, trans. Taipei, Taiwan: Zhiwen Press, 1972.

———. *Zen Buddhism,* Chinese Translation Edition, Men Xiangshen, trans. Taipei, Taiwan: Zhiwen Press, 1975.

——— and Fromm, Erich. *Zen Buddhism and Psychoanalysis.* Chinese Translation Edition, Men Xiangshen, trans. Taipei, Taiwan: Zhiwen Press, 1975.

Tang, Zi-chang. *Wisdom of Dao (Lao Zi: Recompiled, Annotated and Translated).* San Rafael, CA: T.C. Press, 1969.

Taylor, Rodney L. *The Confucian Way of Contemplation (Okada Takehito and the Tradition of Quiet-Sitting).* Columbia, SC: University of South Carolina Press, 1988.

Veith, Ilith, trans. *The Yellow Emperor's Classic of Internal Medicine*. Revised ed. Berkeley, CA: University of California Press, 1972.

Waley, Arthur. *The Way and its Power: A Study of the Tao Te Ching and its Place in Chinese Thought*. 18th Printing. New York: Grove Press, Inc., 1982.

Wang, Yen-nien. *Taichi Quan: Yang Family Hidden Tradition, An Explanation through Photos*. Julia F. Fairchild, trans. Taipei, Taiwan: The Grand Hotel Taichi Chuan Association, 1988.

Watts, Alan. *The Way of Zen*. New York: Vintage Books, 1957.

——. *The Spirit of Zen: A Way of Life, Work and Art in the Far East*. New York: Grove Press, 1958.

——, and Al Chung-liang Huang. *Tao: The Watercourse Way*. New York: Pantheon Books, 1975.

Werner, E.T.C. *Myths and Legends of China*. Reprint. Singapore: Graham Brash (PTE) Ltd., 1985.

Wing, R.L. *The I Ching Workbook*. Wellingborough, UK: The Aquarian Press, 1984.

Wu, John C. H. *The Golden Age of Zen*. Rev. Ed. Taipei, Taiwan: United Publishing Center, 1975.

Wu, Yi. *Zhongyong Zheng de Zhexue* (*The Sincerity Philosophy of The Doctrine of Mean*). Taipei, Taiwan: Dong Da Books, Co., 1976.

——. *Zhexue Jiangyenlu* (*Lectures on Philosophy*). Taipei, Taiwan: Dong Da Books, Co., 1976.

Xie, Huan-zhang, ed. *Qigong de Kexue Jichu* (*Scientific Basis of Qigong*). Beijing: Beijing Ligong University Press, 1988.

Xie, Zhu-fan and Huang, Xiao-kai, eds. *Dictionary of Traditional Chinese Medicine*. Hong Kong: The Commercial Press, Ltd., 1984.

Yan, Johnson F. *The Tao of Biotech*. Federal Way, WA: (Private Publishing), 1987.

Zheng, Manqing and Lin, Pinshi. *Zhonghua Yiyaoxue Shi* (*A History of Traditional Chinese Medicine*). Taipei, Taiwan: Taiwan Commercial Press, 1982.

Zhou, Xue-xi. *Yixue Shiqiang (Ten Lectures on the Study of Yi Jing)*. Chengdu, China: Sichuan Scientific and Technological Press, 1986.

# Index

**129**

# ACCHS

The Academy of Chinese Culture and Health Sciences is a private non-profit graduate college accredited for the Master of Traditional Chinese Medicine degree program. It was founded in Oakland, California in 1983 by Dr. Wei Tsuei, an accomplished practitioner of traditional Chinese medicine, Taichi Chuan, Chi Kung, and meditation. The program features cultivation of the intellect, understanding of human nature, development of critical thinking, and analysis, evaluation and effective clinical practice based on Chiense medical knowledge.

Emphasizing that Chinese philosophy and culture are the roots of Chinese medicine, the program aims to teach students the theory and practice of traditional Chinese medicine in lights of its cultural and philosophiucal basis, with Yin Yang theory at its core. Through the arts of Taichi, Chi Kung and meditation, the Academy nurtures the development of self-awareness and growth in its students.

The Academy plants further seeds for the appreciation of Chinese culture and traditional medicine in the United States through its community outreach, successful clinical programs, cooperative communication with other medical facilities, and promotion of the exchange of medical knowledge.

## ACCHS Series

The ACCHS Series of academic publications aims to cover topics in Chinese culture for all those interested in the Chinese approach to life and healthful living. It includes textbooks on traditional Chinese medicine, research and/or survey books in the realms of Chinese culture, philosophy, Taichi Chuan, Chi Kung, and Taichi meditation.

*Roots of Chinese Culture and Medicine* by Wei Tsuei is the introductory book of the series, providing a foundation for future works. The following are planned topics for forthcoming works in the series:

**Roots of Human Sexuality**
**Roots of Chi Kung**
**The Gate of Taichi Chuan**
**Taichi Meditation**
**No Hangups**
**Traditional Meridian Poems**

**ACCHS**
**420 Fourteenth Street**
**Oakland, California 94612**
**USA**